Physiology
and
Performance

ISBN 0 947850 24 4

Editors
Paul Ledger and Fiona Carpenter

Sub-editors
S Bird, B Davies, A Driver, P Harrison, N Murphy, S Rowell, P Thompson

Typesetter
Catherine Worsley

Illustrator
Jo Willard

sports coach UK would like to thank Richard Godfrey, Alan Lynn and Jenny Roberts
for their valuable input to the 2002 reprint.

Cover photo courtesy of actionplus sports images.

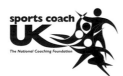

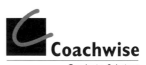

Coachwise Solutions

sports coach UK
114 Cardigan Road
Headingley
Leeds LS6 3BJ
Tel: 0113-274 4802
Fax: 0113-275 5019
E-mail: coaching@sportscoachuk.org
Website: www.sportscoachuk.org

Patron: HRH The Princess Royal

Published on behalf of **sports coach UK** by
Coachwise Solutions
Coachwise Ltd
Chelsea Close
Off Amberley Road
Armley
Leeds LS12 4HP
Tel: 0113-231 1310
Fax: 0113-231 9606
E-mail: enquiries@coachwisesolutions.co.uk
Website: www.coachwisesolutions.co.uk

Why do some performers finish competitions strongly while others tire and fade? How can performers improve strength and speed? Why is flexibility important? These are just some of the questions asked by sports performers and coaches.

This resource is for coaches, teachers, students and performers who want an easy to read introduction to fitness and how the body works. Free of unnecessary jargon, it will help you understand how the body functions, how it is affected by physical activity and how it adapts to the demands of physical activity. It is divided into two sections:

- **Section One** explains the basic structure and function of the body including a chapter on nutrition and the energy systems.

- **Section Two** describes the components of fitness and principles of training, including chapters on endurance, strength, speed, power and flexibility.

To help you work through the book, each chapter includes a number of panels which help you relate material to your own sport. Tasks provide you with the opportunity of applying this knowledge to practical situations. At the end of each chapter a brief summary helps reinforce the key points.

This resource builds on the information and practical application gained in the **sports coach UK** workshop **Fitness and Training.**

Throughout this pack, the pronouns he, she, him, her and so on are interchangeable and intended to be inclusive of both males and females. It is important in sport, as elsewhere, that both genders have equal status and opportunities.

Contents

SECTION TWO: Fitness Components and Training 96

CHAPTER FOUR:
Endurance

CHAPTER FIVE:
Strength, Speed and Power

CHAPTER SIX:
Flexibility

SECTION ONE:
Functional Anatomy, Physiology and Energy Sources

Introduction

This section examines the structure and function of the human body and the sources of energy it utilises for physical performance. An understanding of functional anatomy is essential for anyone involved in sport (coach, teacher or performer) to appreciate how the body moves. Such an understanding is vital in developing effective training programmes and good technique, minimising injuries and optimising performance.

- **Chapter One** will concentrate on basic anatomy covering the bones, joints, levers and muscles of the body. The composition of muscle and the significance of fibre types are examined to enable coaches and performers to understand how the body meets the specific demands of their sport.

- **Chapter Two** examines how the body produces the movements required in sport and physical activity. The chapter helps explain the importance of oxygen and how it is transported and delivered to the working muscles. The role of the heart, lungs and associated elements of the cardio-respiratory system are examined together with the effects of exercise on each.

- **Chapter Three** explains how the body obtains energy from food and converts it to muscle fuel to perform sport or physical activity. Coaches and performers will find this knowledge essential for maximising energy storage and usage during training and competition.

CHAPTER ONE:
Structure of the Body

1.0 Introduction

During the last few decades there has been a noticeable increase in the popularity of sport and physical activity. This is due to the promotion of healthy lifestyles, (particularly at a recreational level), and the increased necessity to be physically fit to perform at a competitive level. To design appropriate training programmes, develop correct technique, minimise the risk of injury and optimise performance, it is important that coaches and performers gain sound knowledge of the structure and function of the skeleton, muscles and joints.

1.1 Functions of the Skeleton

The human skeleton forms the framework of the body and comprises 206 bones of varying shapes and sizes. An appreciation of the functions and structure of the skeleton is fundamental to developing both technique and fitness and in devising training programmes for young people to ensure they take account of the immature skeleton and growing bones.

The skeleton has five basic functions:

- **Support**. Most body tissues and organs are fairly soft and need support. The skeleton provides a solid framework without which the body would be a shapeless mass.

- **Movement**. The bones, joints and muscles form a series of powerful and complex lever systems. These enable the body to move effectively and allow different parts of the body to operate with a high degree of precision and control.

- **Protection**. The body depends upon the coordination of a number of different systems (eg the cardiovascular system), most of which are structurally very delicate and therefore vulnerable to blows, pressure and friction. The framework of the skeleton provides this protection (eg the skull or cranium protects the brain and the ribs or thorax protect the heart and lungs).

- **Blood cell production**. The bone marrow contained within some of the bones produces red blood cells and some white blood cells. The red blood cells are vital for the transport of oxygen through the circulatory system, while the white cells are part of the body's defence against infection.

- **Calcium storage**. Calcium is essential for health. The normal diet provides sufficient calcium for a person's needs. If, however, the body is deprived of calcium, it will temporarily absorb it from the bones, which are largely composed of calcium phosphate. Calcium deficiency is said to be a contributory factor in the development of **osteoporosis.** When calcium intake is less than calcium needs, it is usually taken from the bones resulting in an increased brittleness. In performers, low calcium levels may contribute to a higher incidence of stress fractures.

TASK

Many systems (eg respiratory system) of the body are highly dependent on the bone structure. For example, the bones in the nasal cavity (inside of the nose) form a series of passageways that help clean, moisten and warm inhaled (breathed in) air.

Think how the basic functions of the skeleton relate to your sport.

1.2 Types of Bones

Bones are normally classified according to their shape:

- **Long bones** – the larger bones of the body providing effective levers for movement (eg bone in the thigh – **femur**, the upper arm – **humerus**).
- **Short bones** – small bones which are very strong and well adapted to resist compression forces (eg small bones of the foot – **tarsals**, the wrist – **carpals***).
- **Flat bones** – these bones have a protective function and are often fused together by cartilage for added strength (eg skull, ribs, the iliac bones of the pelvic girdle).
- **Irregular bones** – examples include the vertebrae, which form the spinal column and the facial bones. They provide support and protection.
- **Sesamoid bones** – small oval shaped bones located inside tendons. They are generally found where considerable pressure develops (eg the wrist). The kneecap *(patella)* is the largest example of a sesamoid bone. Its function is unclear but it may improve the leverage of the muscles around the joint and provide additional protection to a vulnerable joint.

1.3 Structure of Bones

A typical long bone consists of a shaft (**diaphysis**) with a bulge called an **epiphysis** at each end (Figure 1). These epiphyses are specially adapted to form joints with the adjacent bones. Between the epiphyses and the diaphysis are the **epiphyseal plates**, where longitudinal growth occurs. In childhood, these areas consist of cartilage which is relatively soft and prone to injury but as the person matures, this cartilage is replaced by bone. There are two types of bone tissue: compact and cancellous (chambered). The diaphysis of a long bone is a tube of compact bone. As the name suggests, this sort of bone is very dense. The tubular construction combines great strength and rigidity with lightness and is able to withstand bending and twisting stresses.

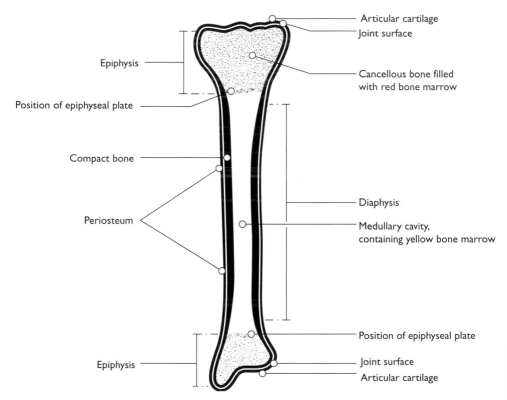

Figure 1: Typical long bone

The epiphyses have a thin outer layer of compact bone and a filling of cancellous bone which is spongy in appearance. This spongy network is designed to cope with the compression forces caused by weight-bearing and the action of the muscles pulling on the bones to cause movement.

The cavity running down the centre of the diaphysis is known as the **medullary cavity**. In adults it contains yellow bone marrow which is a form of fat. The spaces in the cancellous bone are filled with red bone marrow.

The bone is enclosed in a tough skin-like coating (the **periosteum**) except at the surfaces of the epiphyses which form the joint. The periosteum is made up of two layers. The outermost layer is tough connective tissue, the fibres of which actually grow into the underlying compact bone forming a strong inseparable bond. Beneath this is a thin layer containing specialised cells which are vitally important to the growth, repair and remodelling of bones. The periosteum has an abundant nerve and blood supply, and plays an important part in the general nutrition of the bone. Just as the periosteum is intimately fused to the bone, so muscle tendons and ligaments are attached to the periosteum. These connections are so strong that when put under extreme tension, a muscle will very occasionally pull away a flake of bone rather than rupture the connection between the tendon and the periosteum.

Effects of Training

During growth and development, bones will change their size and shape. Physical activity will also stimulate the production of bone tissue to compensate for the stresses placed on it by training. If the intensity of training is too high, damage and injury of the bone can occur (eg shin soreness caused by an inflammation of the periosteum, not the flaking of the bone).

Conversely, reduced stress results in bone tissue **atrophy**, which is a reduction in both the weight and strength of the bone. This is particularly significant following a lay off due to injury. Bone is the slowest of all tissues to recover and it is, therefore, important for performers to return to full training very gradually, to allow the bones to adapt.

Bone growth and the young performer:

Progressive and appropriate exercise programmes must be devised for young performers to protect the growth plates within the skeleton from possible damage. Consider the potential damage that might be inflicted on a young gymnast undergoing intensive training sessions and at the same time, trying to maintain a low body weight. The relentless stress imposed on the joints during jumps, tumbles and handstands can lead to injury and even permanent bone and joint deformation. For example, Osgood Schlatter's condition is seen quite frequently in young, teenage footballers and is an overuse of the tibial tubercle. Exercise programmes need to be modified during the growth period to account for these developments. If you are involved in coaching children, be aware of the training implications on the young body and the measures you can take to prevent injury.

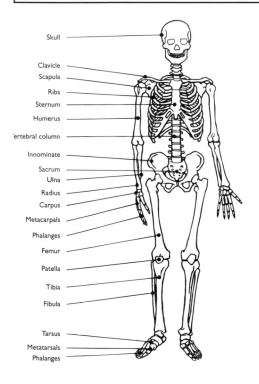

Skull
Clavicle
Scapula
Ribs
Sternum
Humerus
Vertebral column
Innominate
Sacrum
Ulna
Radius
Carpus
Metacarpals
Phalanges
Femur
Patella
Tibia
Fibula
Tarsus
Metatarsals
Phalanges

Figure 2: The human skeleton

1.4 Human Skeleton

The human skeleton (Figure 2) is composed of a complex collection of bones which all have specific roles to play. It can be divided into the:

- axial skeleton (skull, sternum, ribs and spine), forming the centre axis

- appendicular skeleton, consisting of the remaining bones.

The axial skeleton consists of the following:

- **Skull** (cranium), which is made up of a number of interconnecting bones fused together with cartilage. It accommodates and protects the brain and sense organs (eg eyes, inner ear within the skull).

- **Vertebral column** (backbone) which includes 33 vertebrae:

  - Seven cervical vertebrae (neck) including the atlas and axis (top two)

  - Twelve thoracic vertebrae (chest region)

  - Five lumbar vertebrae (lower back)

  - Five sacral vertebrae fused to form the sacrum

  - Four coccygeal vertebrae fused to form the coccyx.

- **Thorax** comprising the breastbone (**sternum**) and twelve pairs of ribs attached to the thoracic vertebrae.

The appendicular skeleton consists of the following:

- **Shoulder girdle** (pectoral) which includes the two shoulder blades (**scapulae**) and the two collar bones (**clavicles**).

- **Hip girdle** (pelvic) which is made up of the ilium, ischium and pubis bones.

- **Upper limbs** which each include the:

  - humerus (upper arm)

  - radius and ulna (lower arm)

  - eight carpals (wrist bones)

  - five metacarpals (hand)

  - fourteen phalanges (fingers).

- Lower limbs which each include the:

  - femur (thigh)

  - tibia and fibula (shin)

  - seven tarsals (ankle)

  - five metatarsals (foot)

  - fourteen phalanges (toes).

TASK

Movements such as throwing a ball and jumping require the coordinated use of bones and muscles. To understand how muscles produce different movements (described in Section 1.14 page 30), you need to know where the bones attach.

Consider the techniques commonly used in your sport. Identify the associated bones and the role each plays (in coordination with the muscles) in executing the required movement.

Structure of a Typical Vertebra

The spine (**vertebral column**) is extremely complex in structure, allowing a combination of flexibility and strength. Additionally it provides the necessary protection to the spinal cord, supports the weight of the upper body and transmits it to the lower limbs (Figure 3).

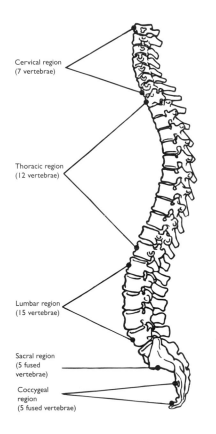

Cervical region
(7 vertebrae)

Thoracic region
(12 vertebrae)

Lumbar region
(15 vertebrae)

Sacral region
(5 fused
vertebrae)

Coccygeal
region
(5 fused vertebrae)

Figure 3: Spinal column

Each vertebra consists of a body to which is attached the **neural arch** (Figure 4).

The arch is made up of two short projections from the back of the body (**pedicles**). Joining the pedicles are two flat plates of bone (**laminae**) which join together in the midline. The vertebral arch encloses a gap (the **vertebral foramen**) in which lies the spinal cord. On each side of the vertebral arch there are two more bony projections called **transverse processes**. These act as short levers for some of the spinal muscles and also as points of attachment for ligaments.

At the junction of the two laminae is the **spinous process**, which projects backwards and serves as a point of attachment for muscles and ligaments. At the point at which the pedicles and laminae join, there are four small joint surfaces. Two of these project upwards and two downwards. In both cases they articulate with similar surfaces on the vertebrae above and below. The size, shape and angle of these articular facets vary in different parts of the spine and this is one of the factors influencing the movements possible in each area.

Between the neural arches of adjacent vertebrae and on each side, there is a small gap (**intervertebral foramen**) at the junction of the pedicles and the bodies of the vertebrae (Figure 4).

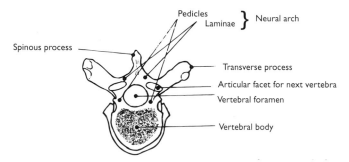

Typical vertebra (front – anterior view)

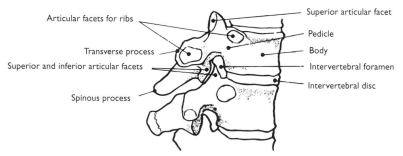

Two vertebrae (side – lateral view)

Figure 4: Typical vertebrae

The spinal nerves, originating from the spinal cord, pass through these gaps on each side of every vertebra.

The bodies of adjacent vertebrae are joined by a pad called an **intervertebral disc**, composed principally of fibro-cartilage with a small amount of jelly-like pulp filling the centre. Trauma to these discs, a degenerative problem, are often blamed for back pain. They are very firmly attached to the vertebral bodies and act as shock absorbers, preventing the skull and brain from being jarred during running or jumping.

The discs, together with the intervertebral joints, allow movement to occur between adjacent vertebrae.

Although the amount of movement possible between any two vertebrae is quite small, the overall movement achieved over the entire spinal column is very large. The discs are thickest in the cervical and lumbar regions, permitting the widest range of mobility. Good spinal mobility is important for most sports and fundamental in activities such as gymnastics.

Nearly 70% of all cricket injuries occur to the back. Some bowlers are susceptible to lower back problems due to a specific fast (action) bowling technique which involves the asymmetric twisting and bending of the spinal vertebrae causing increased stresses on the vertebrae and spinal discs. Coaches must assess the technique of each performer in relation to the design of the skeleton.

The importance of spinal mobility varies between sports. Think how the spine is used in your sport and the possible implications of poor technique.

1.5 Joints

Having an understanding of the joints of the body will help coaches optimise technique, develop good flexibility and help prevent injury. The term **joint articulation** refers to a point of contact between two bones or between cartilage and bones. Some joints permit no movement, others permit slight movement, while others allow a much greater range of movement. Joints are classified according to the degree of movement they permit. The joints are classified as follows:

- **Fibrous** joints are strong, rigid immovable joints. Most joints of this type are sutures (eg joints between the bones of the skull).

- **Cartilaginous** joints which allow slight movement (eg the joints in the spine between the vertebrae and intervertebral discs and the symphysis or the symphysis pubis).

- **Synovial** joints which are freely movable, such as the hips and elbows.

The freely moving synovial joints will be examined in greater detail as these are most important to the sports performer.

1.6 Types of Synovial Joints

Synovial joints can be further classified into six types – ball and socket, hinge, pivot, condyloid, gliding and saddle joints. They are also classified according to their structure and the movement they permit.

Ball and socket joint, which permits the widest range of movement (eg shoulder and hip joints).

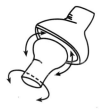

Figure 5: Ball and socket joint

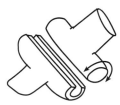

Figure 6: Hinge joint

Hinge joint, which as the name suggests, permits movement in one plane only (eg joints of the fingers, knee and elbow).

Pivot joint, which allows rotational movement (eg the **axis** and **atlas** vertebrae of the neck and the joint between the top of the radius and the ulna).

Figure 7: Pivot joint

Condyloid joint, which allows movement in two planes at right angles to each other (eg wrist joint between the **carpus** and the lower ends of the ulna and radius).

Figure 8: Condyloid joint

Gliding joint, a small joint where movement is limited to short gliding movements, the direction of which depends on the shape of the joint surfaces (eg joints within the **tarsus** and **carpus** bones of the feet and hand respectively).

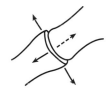

Figure 9: Gliding joint

Saddle joint, like the condyloid joint, permits movement in two planes at right angles to each other (eg the base of the thumb).

Figure 10: Saddle joint

TASK

The joint structures within the body allow certain ranges of limb movement. Each sport will make particular demands on certain joints. For instance, the basketball player requires a wider than normal range of movement within the shoulder joint (ball and socket) and the wrist joint (condyloid) to produce effective passing and shooting techniques.

Think about the particular joints used in your sport and identify them according to their structure and function. A coach needs to be aware of the potential range of movement of these joints to improve technique and prevent injury.

1.7 Structure of a Synovial Joint

Although optimal joint mobility is essential to high level performance, it is often neglected in training. It is important to have a thorough understanding of the basic structure of synovial joints and the factors affecting both mobility and the potential range of movement. Figure 11 illustrates the typical features of a synovial joint.

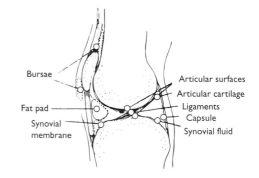

Side – lateral view

Joint surface

These are shaped to accept each other, the exact fit depending on the type and function of the joint. For example, the hip joint has a large deep socket which is the right size to take the ball-like head of the femur. The result is a joint combining a good range of movement with good stability, which explains why hip

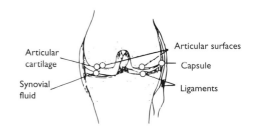

Front – anterior view

Figure 11: Typical synovial joint (knee joint)

dislocations are rare in sport. The surfaces of the joint are covered with a layer of smooth hyaline cartilage (**articular cartilage**) providing a low-friction surface which is very hard-wearing. However, in the shoulder joint the two bones (scapula and humerus) are not as tightly bound as in the hip joint and shoulder injuries are common due to shoulder instability.

Joint capsule

The epiphyses of the bones on each side of a joint are held together by the joint capsule which plays an important part in maintaining joint stability. It is composed of tough white fibrous tissue which merges with the periosteum of the bones resulting in a strong, stretch-resistant structure.

Ligaments

Ligaments are strong bands of white fibrous tissue which run between the ends of the bones forming the joint. Ligaments can exist either as a well-defined thickening in the joint capsule or as independent structures situated outside (or sometimes inside) the joint space to provide stability. They are frequently damaged in the ankle and knee joints during physical activity. Permanent instability in the joint may result if the ligaments are severely torn.

As they are poorly supplied by blood vessels, recovery from injury is often slow.

> It is estimated that injuries to soft tissue (eg muscle, tendons) take about one year to recover fully and regain their initial strength and resilience. Even when there is no longer pain and the full range of movement has been re-established, specific stretching and strengthening exercises to the damaged area should continue for about 12 months to avoid recurring injury.

Synovial Membrane and Fluid

Lining the inside of the capsule is the synovial membrane which has an abundance of specialised cells which secrete synovial fluid. Synovial fluid acts as a lubricant and provides nourishment for articular cartilage. As exercise begins, synovial fluid is absorbed into the articular cartilage (Figure 11 on page 12) covering the ends of the bones, causing it to thicken and improve cushioning between the bones. An increase in temperature makes the fluid less sticky and improves joint mobility. As the joint cools (eg after exercise) the thin film of synovial fluid on the hyaline cartilage disappears. This indicates the importance of warm-up and cool-down. Training will cause a thickening of the hyaline cartilage so the joint can tolerate greater forces. If a joint is damaged and the synovial membrane becomes inflamed, the amount of fluid in the joint cavity increases resulting in swelling and tenderness.

TASK

A thorough warm-up is important before all sports to prepare the body for action and help prevent joint damage and muscle strain. It would be hard to envisage 100 metre sprinters walking straight onto the track, recording fast times and remaining injury free. However, it may be more difficult to accept that an archer or curler needs an adequate warm-up but this is equally important to increase the flow of synovial fluid to lubricate and prevent friction within the joint.

Think about an injury you or another performer have experienced that can be related to an inadequate warm-up. Are the warm-up routines you use sport specific? What changes could make them more effective?

Some joints also have the following additional structures:

- **Cartilage** of varying shapes (eg in knee and shoulder joint). This improves stability, reduces friction and pressure on the articular cartilage and helps absorb shock. It often slightly expands in size during warm-up which increases joint stability.

- **Bursae** are small flat sacs made of white fibrous tissue and lined with a synovial membrane, which secretes fluid into the free space within the bursa. They are found in most of the major joints and serve to reduce friction (eg between tendons and bone, between two muscle tendons, and sometimes between bone and skin). Frictional bursitis resulting in swelling and pain can occur in performers who are subjected to repetitive movements (eg tennis players). Bursitis frequently affects joints in the shoulder, elbow, hip, knee and around the heel.

- **Fat pads** exist around the joint margins to accommodate the changing spaces caused by movement of the joint. Although they are firmly anchored, they can become momentarily trapped resulting in painful inflammation.

Cartilage injuries of the knee often result from excessive, repeated, direct impact situations (eg long jumping, gymnastics, triple jumping, weight lifting). Injuries to the articular cartilage surfaces of the knee joint can also affect the joint surfaces of the femur, tibia and patella. Cartilage damage can result in large cracks in the joint surface and continued degeneration may lead to premature **osteoarthritis**. Coaches and performers should be aware of the symptoms (swelling and pain of the joint) and obtain medical treatment. Training programmes and technique should be closely monitored to avoid potentially dangerous exercises.

1.8 Types of Movement

Each joint has its own characteristic range and type of movement. A knowledge of these movements is essential in the development of efficient and safe technique. The following definitions refer to movements made from the **anatomical position** (ie standing with palms of the hands facing forward, feet and head facing forwards).

An explanation of the types of movement possible is provided in Table 1.

Table 1: Classification of movements

Flexion:	reducing the angle at a joint (eg bending a limb).
Extension:	increasing the angle at a joint (eg straightening a limb).
Horizontal flexion:	flexes limb across midline of body.
Abduction:	movement of a limb away from midline of body.
Adduction:	movement of a limb towards midline of body.
Internal rotation:	circular movement of limb towards body.
External rotation:	circular movement of limb away from body.
Circumduction:	one end of a limb (at the point of origin) remains almost stable while the other end (furthest from point of origin) moves in a circle.
Plantar flexion:	extending the foot away from the body.
Dorsiflexion:	pulling the foot up towards the shin.
Inversion/eversion:	allows foot to tilt from side to side from ankle.
Supination:	complex movement of hand to face palm upwards.
Pronation:	complex movement of hand to face palm downwards.

To understand the type and range of movement available, it may help to try the movements of each joint physically as they are described in the following pages. Consider the demands of your own sport as you read through the different joints.

Shoulder Joint

This is the most mobile joint in the body. The very large range of movement is really a combination of shoulder joint and shoulder girdle movement.

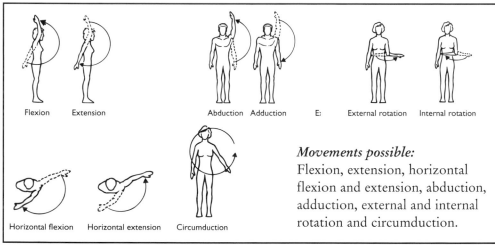

Movements possible:
Flexion, extension, horizontal flexion and extension, abduction, adduction, external and internal rotation and circumduction.

Figure 12: Shoulder movements

Elbow Joint

The elbow joint is a hinge joint.

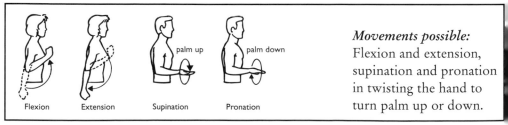

Movements possible:
Flexion and extension, supination and pronation in twisting the hand to turn palm up or down.

Figure 13: Elbow movements

Wrist and Finger Joints

The wrist joint is a condyloid joint. The finger joints are hinge joints.

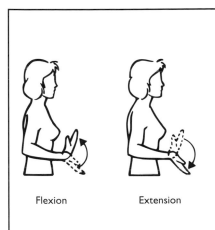

Flexion   Extension

Movements possible:
Flexion and extension. The wrist can also move slightly from side to side (known as ulna and radial deviation). The metacarpal/phalangeal joints of the hand are also capable of abduction and adduction. The thumb has a far greater range of movement than the fingers. Not only can it flex and extend but it can also move away from and towards the midline of the hand (abduct and adduct). The movement of bringing the tip of the thumb across to the base of the little finger contributes greatly to manual dexterity.

Figure 14: Wrist and finger movements

Hip Joint

Being a ball and socket joint, the hip joint enjoys a wide range of mobility. The stability requirement of the joint makes its range of movement less free than the shoulder but the types of movement are similar.

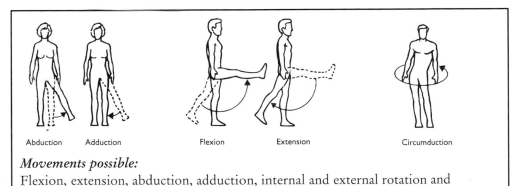

Abduction   Adduction   Flexion   Extension   Circumduction

Movements possible:
Flexion, extension, abduction, adduction, internal and external rotation and circumduction.

Figure 15: Hip movements

Knee Joint

The knee joint is essentially a hinge joint.

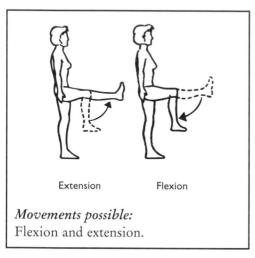

Extension   Flexion

Movements possible:
Flexion and extension.

Figure 16: Knee movements

Ankle Joint

This is a true hinge joint.

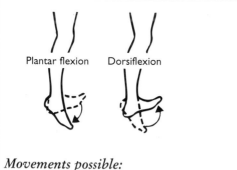

Plantar flexion   Dorsiflexion

Movements possible:
Plantar flexion (the downward movement of the foot), dorsiflexion (the opposite movement).

Figure 17: Ankle movements

Mid-tarsal Joints

These are gliding joints.

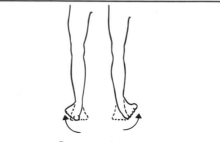

Eversion   Inversion
(both diagrams show the right leg and foot from the front)

Movements possible:
Supination and **pronation** (allowing the foot to tilt from side to side). Supination may also be referred to as **inversion** or **adduction**, while pronation may also be referred to as **eversion** or **abduction**.

Figure 18: Mid-tarsal movements

Spinal Movements

Although the actual amount of movement possible between two adjacent vertebrae is limited, the total movement of the whole vertebral column is quite considerable. The overall movements are flexion, extension, lateral flexion, rotation and circumduction but not all parts of the spine are capable of these movements to the same degree.

Movements possible

- **Flexion** occurs in the cervical spine, some in the lumbar region and very little in the thoracic area.

- **Extension** is quite free in the cervical and lumbar regions but very limited in the thoracic spine.

- **Lateral flexion** takes place in all parts of the spine but is most marked in the cervical and lumbar regions.

- **Rotation** is good in the cervical and upper thoracic regions but minimal in the lumbar region.

These are shown in Figure 19.

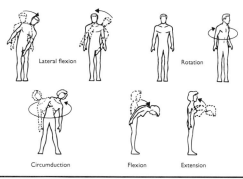

Figure 19: Spinal movements

TASK

In every sport, technical improvements can be made if the joints are used in the correct sequence and with the appropriate timing. Coaches and performers need to analyse the joint movement and muscle action of techniques to ensure an efficient technique is developed safely and effectively. Think about the javelin thrower and the action at the major joints and associated muscles at the point of release of the javelin. You may find it useful to break down action in your sport in terms of joint, action and major muscles:

Joint	Action	Major muscles[1]
Shoulder	First flexion	Shoulder (deltoid)
	Second flexion	Chest (pectorals)

Analyse a specific movement in your sport in the same way. This type of analysis should help in skill development and appropriate strength training to help improve performance and reduce the risk of joint injuries.

---

1   The muscular system will be described in Section 1.11 page 23

1.9 Factors Affecting Joint Mobility

Several factors influence the potential range of movement in any given joint:

- Shape and fit of the joint surfaces
- Bony structures around the joint
- Joint structures
- Temperature
- Limiting effect of the muscles
- Age
- Gender.

These will all be considered in the following sections.

Shape and Fit of the Joint Surfaces

Obviously the shape of the joint surfaces and the degree to which they accept each other will determine the type and range of movement. For example, the socket of the shoulder joint is quite flat and small, and therefore makes only a small amount of contact with the ball of the humerus. This allows a large range of movement but at the expense of joint stability, which is why the joint is relatively easily dislocated. By contrast, the shape of the humerus and ulna of the elbow joint permits movement in one plane only, limiting mobility but improving stability.

Bony Structures around the Joint

There are situations where bone-to-bone contact prevents any further movement in a joint. For example, the spinous processes of the thoracic vertebrae lock together when this area of the spine is fully extended. At the elbow joint, the projection on the ulna (olecranon process) locks against the humerus when fully extended, preventing excessive movement of the elbow joint.

Joint Structures

The joint capsule and ligaments prevent undue movement which could lead to damage. Muscle bulk can occasionally limit full range of movement (eg in full knee flexion when the calf and back of the thigh come into contact). Occasionally, the tension of the skin itself can limit the range of movement. With constant mobilising work, the skin stretches and evidence of this may be left as stretch marks in the skin.

Temperature

Gymnasts and short-event performers who prefer to train and compete in a warm environment, will appreciate it is easier to mobilise a joint when it is warm. At ambient temperatures above 43°C (110°F), it is possible to obtain a

20% increase in mobility compared with normal room temperature (about 21°C, 70°F). As temperatures fall below this, mobility is progressively reduced. An effective warm-up would include an extended period of large muscle group activity to raise body temperature, followed by mobilising exercises for all the joints to be used. The stretching of muscle tissue should only take place when the joint has been fully mobilised.

Limiting Effect of the Muscles

A trained muscle has the tendency to shorten if not fully stretched after exercise which can reduce joint mobility. To ensure flexibility gains are achieved (Chapter Six) throughout the full range of movement, it is important to include regular stretching exercises, especially if strength, power or speed training are involved (Section 5.9 page 125).

Age and Gender

Research shows that younger people are able to respond more readily to mobilising activity than older people who use extremes of joint range less frequently. Regular mobility work will help to maintain joint range. It has also been shown that women tend to be more flexible than men, which may be due to anatomical differences as the flexibility variation is greater after puberty. It has been suggested that athletes who have

suffered from persistent joint injuries are more susceptible to osteoarthritis in later life. However, there has been no evidence to date to indicate that athletes suffer more than sedentary people.

TASK

Extend the elbow joint and note how the movement is restricted by the bony contact between the upper (humerus) and lower arm (radius and ulna). Certain joints are of particular importance to given sports (eg the knee joint in soccer is prone to stressful movement, shoulder movement in gymnastics is essential to mobility). Think about the stress placed on these joints during activity that acts against normal structure and function of the joint (eg soccer players often suffer damage to the slightly movable joint at the front of the pelvis due to constant use of one-legged jumps and landings).

Try to think of specific joints prone to stress from a particular technique in your sport.

1.10 Lever Systems of the Body

The bones of the skeleton act as levers and are rotated about the joints by the muscles to produce the range of movements required in physical activity. The coach and performer will need to have a basic understanding of the mechanics involved to ensure the development of effective and efficient technique and so reduce the likelihood of injury and fatigue. Levers can be classified according to the relative position of the:

- **fulcrum** (axis) about which the turning occurs

- point where **force** is applied

- point of **resistance.**

There are three classes of musculoskeletal levers in the body:

- First class levers

- Second class levers

- Third class levers.

First class levers (Figure 20) are those where the fulcrum is located between the point of force and point of resistance (eg skull rotating on top of the vertebral column, action of the muscles at the back of the upper arm (**triceps**) to operate the elbow).

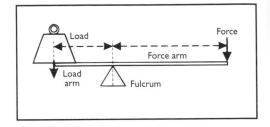

Figure 20: First class levers

Second class levers (Figure 21) are those where the point of resistance is positioned between the fulcrum and the point of application. Examples found in the body are rare and controversial although some are generally accepted as accurate (eg the lower calf muscle, **gastrocnemius** in the action of flexing the knee, lowering action of the jaw bone in chewing action). As the force arm is always longer than the resistance arm, the amount of force applied will increase at the expense of range and speed of movement.

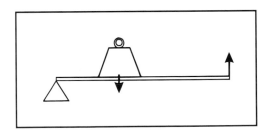

Figure 21: Second class levers

1   If you are unsure of the location of certain muscles, refer to Figure 25 page 32.

Third class levers (Figure 22) are those where the point of force is positioned between the fulcrum and the point of resistance. Most of the musculoskeletal levers in the body are third class. As the force arm is always shorter, both range and speed of movement are enhanced at the expense of the force exerted (eg shoulder muscle – deltoid action in raising arm, upper arm muscle – brachialis in elbow flexion). Many sport implements (eg bats, racquets, golf clubs, hockey sticks) act as third class levers and therefore further increase the potential for range and speed of movement.

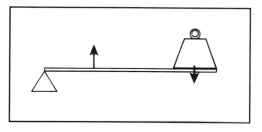

Figure 22: Third class levers

The coach and performer should be aware of the individual differences in attachment points of various muscle groups (eg biceps, deltoid, pectorals) which help to explain why certain performers possess a mechanical advantage in particular skills. The forces exerted must be in excess of the load to produce movement. The relative lengths of the force and load – arms in human levers mean that the muscles nearly always generate forces far in excess of the loads being moved.

Identification of the lever systems used in specific sports will assist in the analysis of skills and development of appropriate and effective coaching programmes.

1.11 Muscular System

There are three types of **muscle** found in the human body:

- **Cardiac muscle** which is highly specialised and found only in the heart.

- **Smooth muscle** which is controlled involuntarily and is found in the digestive tract, circulatory system and respiratory system.

- **Skeletal muscle** is specialised for contraction and may be controlled voluntarily. It can also occur as a reflex response, ie a fast involuntary contraction (such as the knee jerk).

1 If you are unsure of the location of certain muscles, refer to Figure 25 page 32.

1.12 Structure of Skeletal Muscle

Skeletal muscle exerts the force to create the movements required in most sporting situations (some movements are caused by gravity). A knowledge of the structure of muscles is vital to coaches and performers of all sports to ensure techniques are developed effectively and safely, and strength is optimised.

Structure

Muscle is composed of:

- **contractile tissue** so it can contract

- **connective tissue** to bind it together

- **nerves** so that messages can be sent from the brain and spinal cord to the muscles and from the muscles back to the brain and spinal cord (**central nervous system**)

- **blood vessels** to bring oxygen, remove waste products, supply energy and maintain fluid levels.

Each muscle is composed of many thousands of muscle fibres. The fibres are specialised (muscle) cells which are long, narrow and cylindrical. These fibres lie parallel to one another and range from 10–100 µm in diameter and vary in length. Each fibre is surrounded by a connective tissue sheath called the **endomysium** which is enclosed within the **sarcolemma**. The fibres are bound together in a bundle (**fasciculus**) and wrapped in a connective tissue sheath (**perimysium**).

The connective tissue covering the whole muscle (the epimysium) has a number of functions:

- It **transmits** the force created by the fibres to the ends of the muscles. At the end, the connective tissue comes together to form the tendon which attaches the muscle to the bone. Connective tissue can also form broad sheets (**aponeurosis**), which serve the same function as tendons but connect over a larger area, not at a distinct point.

- It **protects** the more delicate muscle tissue from damage.

A single fibre is composed of a number of **myofibrils**, which in turn contain filaments of the contractile proteins, **myosin** and **actin**. The actual muscle contraction takes place by the rapid transmission of contraction impulses in each muscle fibre. The **sarcomere** is the distance between the linked ends of the actin strands which form a regular pattern along the full length of the muscle fibre (Figure 23).

The **mitochondria** (specialised organelles) are located within the muscle fibres and play a central role in the aerobic production of Adenosine Triphosphate (ATP).

The contraction of muscle is caused by the interaction of the two protein filaments which make up a large proportion of the muscle mass. These two protein filaments, actin and myosin, connect with one another to form cross bridges. This action is repeated many times down each filament across the entire muscle, involving millions of protein filaments. This shortening of the muscle results in the creation of force. This process can be seen more clearly in Figure 24.

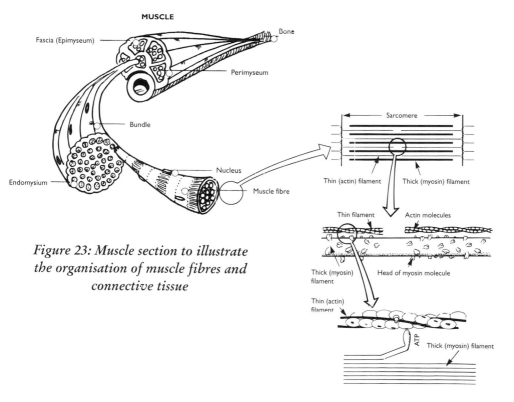

Figure 23: Muscle section to illustrate the organisation of muscle fibres and connective tissue

Figure 24: Small section of a muscle fibre showing the actin and myosin filaments

TASK

Muscle fibre length varies with both muscle size and its function. For instance, the eye muscles, needed for rapid and precise movement, consist of shorter fibres and measure up to one tenth of a millimetre (mm) in length. In contrast, the larger leg muscles needed for strength and endurance consist of fibres up to 40mm in length. Increases in muscle size depend on the type of training (eg weight training) involved, and are due to the growth in diameter of the individual fibres (hypertrophy). Current research has shown that increases in muscle size may also be due to individual fibres dividing to form new fibres, therefore increasing the number of fibres (hyperplasia).

Consider the muscular demands in your sport and compare them with related or differing sports (eg the site and size of muscular development in downhill skiers compared with freestyle wrestlers).

Nerves

For a skeletal muscle fibre to contract, a stimulus must be applied to it. The stimulus is delivered by a nerve cell, or a neuron. A **neuron** has a threadlike process called a fibre, or axon, that may run 91cm or more to a muscle. A bundle of such fibres from many different neurons composes a nerve. A neuron that stimulates muscle tissue is called a **motor neurone** (Figure 25).

Afferent nerves transmit messages to the central nervous system (CNS) and **efferent nerves** transmit messages from the CNS. Impulses pass in both directions within the nervous system communicating between the brain and the rest of the body. However, each neurone transmits in one direction only, allowing changes in the environment to be detected and the appropriate responses made (eg a muscle contraction in order to kick a ball).

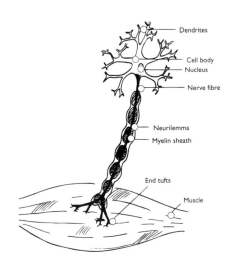

Figure 25: Structure of a motor neurone

The decision to move is made in a specific area of the brain (**motor cortex**).

The motor cortex receives impulses from a wide range of sense organs throughout the body (eg visual receptors, tendon proprioceptors – **golgi tendon organs**, specialised organs within muscles – **muscle spindles**), and the response generated will depend on the information received. Each nerve cell is connected to a number of muscle cells (fibres) to form a **motor unit**.

A nerve cell is usually connected to more than one muscle cell; the actual number depending on the function of the muscle. If fine control is required, one nerve cell will connect with only a few muscle fibres (eg in the eyes where accuracy is important). In muscles which are used for larger movements (eg quadriceps – the muscle in the front part of the thigh), one nerve cell will connect with numerous muscle fibres as less fine control is needed. The muscle as a whole can have graded contractions. The interplay between the CNS to muscle via efferent nerves, the proprioceptors to CNS via afferent nerves, and the subsequent recruitment of motor units determine the force of contraction and the regulation of that force.

During a contraction, the many motor units that make up an entire muscle will contract and relax simultaneously. Therefore the principle does not mean that the entire muscle must be either fully relaxed or fully contracted. The strength of a contraction may be decreased by fatigue, lack of nutrients or lack of oxygen.

The nerve fibre is the projection out from the cell body and its length will vary according to location (eg nerve fibres pass from the cell body contained within the spinal cord, as far as the fingers and toes). The nerve cell membrane (**neurilemma**) and the fatty insulation around it (**myelin sheath**) are responsible for the electrical activity in nerves and the speed of conduction.

TASK

Identify situations in your sport which rely on rapid and efficient responses by the brain to initiate muscle action (eg a cricketer successfully catching the ball during play or a boxer reacting to avoid a punch).

Fibre Types

Skeletal muscle fibres do not all have the same biochemical and physical characteristics. The type and quantity of each muscle fibre type is genetically predetermined. However, the size and metabolic capacities of the muscle can be markedly improved with long-term training.

There are generally considered to be three main types of skeletal muscle fibre:

- **Type I fibres** (red, slow twitch or slow oxidative fibres) contract and relax slowly (but still many times a second) and are resistant to fatigue. Their capacity for slow aerobic work makes them important for aerobic endurance activities such as distance running, cycling or swimming. Successful marathon runners, for example, have a high proportion of these fibres.

- **Type IIa fibres** (white, fast twitch, or fast oxidative glycotic) have a mixed capacity and can work *aerobically* and *anaerobically* (with or without the presence of oxygen). They have less aerobic endurance capacity than the slow twitch fibres but more than the fast glycolytic fibres. These fibres contribute to about 20% of the total and appear to change their characteristics in response to different training programmes.

- **Type IIb fibres** (white, fast twitch or fast glycolytic) are capable of contracting twice as fast as slow twitch fibres, producing very high forces of short duration, but they fatigue quickly. Their capacity for anaerobic work makes them important for sprint activities. Top class sprinters have a high proportion of these fibres.

Further information on the respective contributions of such fibres and their sporting significance is given in Chapter Five.

TASK

Muscle action in all sports requires a contribution from each muscle fibre type. In cricket and long jump, the fast twitch fibres are vital to achieve the rapid reactions and explosive power often needed by performers. Triathletes and marathon canoeists rely more heavily on the slow twitch fibres to sustain performance over long periods of activity. In contrast, soccer and squash players will utilise both types at different times within the game.

Think about the balance of muscle fibres required in your sport and the significance of their overall distribution in the body on determining a performer's potential (eg sprinters have high percentages of fast twitch fibres and low percentages of slow twitch fibres).

Muscle Fibre Recruitment

A muscle contains a collection of motor units (ie consisting of one nerve and all the muscle fibres it stimulates). At rest there will be a small number of motor units working to maintain the tone of the muscle. As the level of activity increases, more and more are recruited. The number of muscle fibres recruited depends partly on information from the sense organs (eg vision and hearing) and partly on the degree of familiarity with the task. The decision to move is made by the motor cortex (part of the brain), while the fine tuning is controlled by an organ beneath the rear part of the cortex (cerebellum). Sense organs supplying information to the cerebellum include the eyes, receptors in tendons (golgi tendon organs) and specialised organs within muscles which detect a change in length (muscle spindles).

To develop an effective training programme, coaches should be aware of the fibre types required in their sport and how they are recruited. There is a general pattern in the order of recruitment of motor units. Generally slow twitch fibres are used to create most of the force in low intensity activity (eg jogging), whereas fast twitch fibres contribute to most of the movement in high intensity activities (eg weight lifting). This recruitment pattern is referred to as the *Size Principle.*

Muscles are highly versatile. For example, in golf the same muscles initiate all the fairway shots, from the drive, off the tee, to the pitch and run. The same muscles might operate within different events but the speed of contraction and muscle fibre recruitment will differ. This depends on the type of movement involved. For example, comparing the use of the thigh muscles (quadriceps and hamstrings) by a long distance runner and a sprinter or comparing the type of muscle action needed to execute an explosive jump to catch a ball, with that of a standing catch.

1.13 Attachment of Muscles

Muscles are attached to bones by tendons and usually run between two bones crossing a joint. Many muscles have points of attachment on more than two bones and cross more than one joint (eg the biceps crosses the shoulder and elbow joint; the hamstrings in the back of the upper leg cross the hip and knee joint). When a muscle contracts, both ends of the muscle are pulled towards each other producing movement at the joint or joints it crosses. In practice, one end of the muscle tends to be fixed (the **origin**) so that the other end moves towards the fixed end (the **insertion**). A general knowledge of the position of a muscle and the direction in which it pulls is needed to analyse and understand movement in sport.

Coaches working with young performers should remember:

- their muscles and nerves are still immature, therefore reaction times are slower and movements may not be refined

- their muscles are not developed sufficiently to lift their own body weight

- the resistance caused by the child's own body is often sufficient to promote improvement.

1.14 Types of Muscle Action

Muscles can be arranged into groups according to the contribution they make to a particular movement. The groups that produce the movement are the:

- **agonist** or **prime movers** which make the greatest contribution to the movement

- **assistant movers or synergists** which, because of their small size or disadvantageous angle of pull, assist the movement

- **antagonists** which relax as the agonists contract (ie they could oppose the particular movement).

There are other ways in which muscle groups cooperate to bring about controlled movement. Often when a muscle contracts, it produces secondary, unwanted movements which must be controlled by groups of muscles. There are two groups of muscle which have this function:

- **Stabilisers and fixators**, which work to stabilise the ends of other muscles so they work effectively.

- **Neutraliser muscles**, which neutralise secondary movements by working in cooperation with the stabilisers.

An example of both stabiliser and neutraliser muscles occurs during contraction of the upper arm (biceps) in elbow flexion. The upper arm is stabilised by the shoulder (deltoid) muscle, while the forearm (brachialis) muscle neutralises the tendency to turn the palm up as the elbow flexes. All muscles act by contraction (ie the muscle fibres contract in order to exert a force) which generates tension in the muscle. However, this does not always mean that the muscle shortens overall – that depends on the load that the muscle is opposing. It is possible to produce an action (**isometric**) where tension is generated but no shortening of the muscle occurs, and to produce an action where tension is generated and the muscle lengthens. The major muscles are shown in Figures 25 and 26.

There are three types of muscular contraction:

- Isotonic action (concentric and eccentric)

- Isometric action

- Isokinetic action.

Isotonic Action
(Iso = same, tonic = tension)

In this type of contraction, the muscle develops tension to overcome a resistance, resulting in the movement of body parts. It is the most familiar type of contraction and is further classified by the action of the muscle fibres exerting a given force:

- **Concentric action** – the muscle shortens and thickens as the insertion moves towards the origin and the joint angle decreases (eg biceps curl – as the weight is lifted towards the chest, the flexors of the elbow joint shorten).

- **Eccentric action** – the muscle lengthens as tension develops. The origin and insertion are pulled apart as the muscle resists the movement (eg lowering the weight in the biceps curl). The quadriceps muscles of the thigh work eccentrically in running, resisting the tendency of the knee joint to buckle each time the foot lands in the running stride.

Isometric Action
(Iso = same, metric = length)

Isometric contractions do not produce movement of the joint but the muscle does develop tension. This is very common and can be seen when an attempt is made to move or lift an immovable object. Isometric contractions occur constantly in all sports, to provide postural stability for those parts of the body not specifically involved in the sport itself.

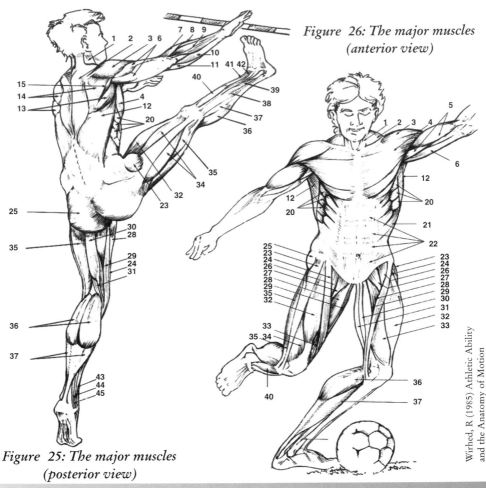

Figure 26: The major muscles (anterior view)

Figure 25: The major muscles (posterior view)

Wirhed, R (1985) Athletic Ability and the Anatomy of Motion

Key to Figures 25 and 26			
1. Sterno-cleido-mastoid	10. Extensor carpi ulnaris	22. Rectus abdominis	34. Vastus lateralis
2. Trapezius	11. Flexor carpi ulnaris	23. Tensor fascia latae	35. Biceps femoris
3. Deltoid	12. Latissimus dorsi	24. Sartorius	36. Gastrocnemius
4. Pectoralis major	13. Teres major	25. Gluteus maximus	37. Soleus
5. Biceps brachii	14. Infraspinatus	26. Illiopsoas	38. Peroneus longus
6. Triceps brachii	15. Teres minor	27. Pectineus	39. Peroneus brevis
7. Brachioradialis	16. Supraspinatus	28. Adductor longus	40. Tibialis anterior
8. Extensor carpi radialis longus and brevis	17. Rhomboid major	29. Gracillis	41. Extensor hallucis longus
	18. Rhomboid minor	30. Semitendinosus	42. Extensor digitorum longus
	19. Levator scapulae	31. Semimembranosus	43. Tibialis posterior
9. Extensor digitorum	20. Serratus anterior	32. Rectus femoris	44. Flexor hallucis longus
	21. External oblique	33. Vastus medialis	45. Flexor digitorum

TASK

To appreciate the way muscles work together, it might help to carry out a press-up, breaking the action down into three stages (but ensure you have warmed-up first). Start facing the ground, hands shoulder width apart, feet or knees resting on the floor.

1 Raise the body off the floor by extending the elbow joints.

2 Hold the position midway with elbows fixed at approximately 90°.

3 Lower the body back to the floor by reversing the action.

Initially the muscle at the back of the upper arm (triceps) will work to extend the elbow joint by shortening. Holding the position midway will result in the triceps and the front of the upper arm (biceps) acting under tension but not changing length (isometric action). Finally on lowering the body under gravity, the triceps control the movement of the body by lengthening under tension (eccentric contraction).

It will be helpful to identify the major movements used in your sport. This should influence the general content of your training programme. Remember to do a thorough warm-up before any physical activity (remember this point when asked to perform any physical tasks throughout this book).

Isokinetic Action
(Iso = same, kinetic = motion)

This refers to muscular contraction at a constant speed over the full range of movement. In order to execute an isokinetic contraction, specialised machines and weight training apparatus are required which provide a resistance equal to the force being applied by the performer throughout the full range of movement. Although isokinetic contractions do not occur in human activity, they are thought to be an effective way of improving muscular strength and have a particular role to play in rebuilding strength following injury.

1.15 Coordination of Opposing Muscle Forces

A high degree of coordination must exist between opposing muscle groups for efficient movement. For example to bend the elbow rapidly, the triceps (antagonist) must relax so that the biceps (agonist) can flex without being impeded.

Group Action of Muscles

Movement is rarely produced as the result of the contraction of only one muscle. Muscles almost invariably act in groups but the contribution of each muscle can vary considerably. This is determined by the level of effort being made, the relative size of the muscles involved and the angle of pull of each muscle. If a movement is being made against a small resistance, then some muscles may make little or no contribution at all. Conversely in a maximal effort, every muscle in the group will make a contribution. For example, when the elbow is flexed, the principal muscles in the group are (in order of importance) brachialis, biceps and brachio-radialis (Figures 25 and 26, page 32). When the effort is low, the force required will easily be provided by the brachialis, with a lesser contribution from the biceps and perhaps nothing from the brachio-radialis. However, if a maximal effort is needed, all three muscles will be working to capacity and other muscles will be used even though their contribution is minimal.

1.16 Range of Movement

Muscles can cause the joint to move from full flexion to full extension. This is called the range of movement and is divided into three parts:

- **Inner range** – the last third of the movement, when the muscle is almost fully contracted and working at its shortest length.
- **Middle range** – the middle third of the movement, when the muscle is neither at its shortest nor longest length. The middle third is the range

which can cause most difficulty because the leverage is unfavourable (eg weight-lifting).

- **Outer range** – the first third of the movement, when the muscle begins the movement and is at its greatest length.

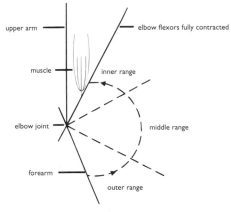

Figure 27: Conventional divisions of joint range for the elbow joint

TASK

A weightlifter carrying out squats with heavy weights is more likely to fail when the knee is at right angles (middle range) as this is where the joint is at its greatest disadvantage. In order to improve, the coach must ensure the training programme compensates for the weak points in any given muscle action.

Think about how this applies to certain moves requiring muscular strength in your sport. Would you expect to follow the same programme as the weightlifter to improve performance?

1.17 Analysis of Muscular Action

In coaching, it is often useful to analyse the muscular work used in the basic techniques of a particular event. By identifying the principal muscle groups involved, it will be easier to devise specific conditioning programmes. It is not necessary to make the analysis too detailed and complicated; only to establish the major muscle groups involved using a systematic approach. This could be done using the following format:

1 Identify the major joints involved and the associated range of movements (drawing simple stick figures can help).

2 Once the movements have been determined, identify the muscles which are involved. Muscles always work in groups to stabilise and neutralise unwanted secondary movements caused by the prime and assistant movers.

For example, the muscles (and their actions) involved in the downswing action of a golfer to the point of contact with the ball have been identified in Table 2.

Apart from conditioning the prime movers, it is also necessary to strengthen the other muscles actively involved in the group action to ensure optimal muscle development and balance.

Table 2: Analysis of the muscular actions involved in the downswing action of a golfer to the point of contact with the ball

Joint	Muscle	Action
Wrist	Wrist flexors	Isometric action to grip the club
Finger	Finger flexors	Isometric action to grip the club
Vertebrae	Lower back (left) (latissimus dorsi)	Concentric action to draw left arm down to point of contact with ball
Vertebrae	Spine (erector spinae)	Stabilising action to prevent flexion of the spine

1.18 Summary

An understanding and basic knowledge of the structure and function of bones, joints, levers and muscles will enable coaches to:

- analyse and teach effective technique
- reduce the risk of injury
- design and develop sound training programmes.

It is important to consider all the physiological and anatomical factors influencing the amount of force that can be generated by a muscle in order to optimise efficiency and improve performance. The following books contain greater detail:

*Farrally, M (2003) **An introduction to the structure of the body.** Leeds, **sports coach UK** and **sport**scotland. ISBN 1 902523 49 0

Gray, H (2002) **Grays Anatomy.** London, Grange Books. ISBN 1 840134 58 5

Palastanga, N, Field, D and Soames, R (2002) **Anatomy and human movement.** London, Butterworth. ISBN 0 750652 41 1

Roberts, J and Faulkener, S (1992) **Biomechanics: problem solving for functional activity.** London, C V Mosby. ISBN 0 8016 8979 1

Seeley, D and Stephens, R (2002) **Anatomy and physiology.** London, C V Mosby. ISBN 0 071150 90 0

Wirhed, R (1997) **Athletic ability and the anatomy of motion.** London, Wolfe Medical. ISBN 0 723426 43 0

* Available from **Coachwise 1st4sport** (tel 0113-201 5555) or visit www.1st4sport.com

TASK

The following tasks will help you assess your knowledge and understanding of the structure and function of the skeleton, joints and muscles and relate this to your specific sport. Use the diagrams provided in this chapter to help you analyse the joints and muscle groups used and identify how this can help improve technique and performance.

1   Identify the major movements used in your sport and the associated joints. Slowly repeat these movements (if possible in front of a mirror):

   •   To what extent is the structure limiting its potential for movement?

   •   What structural limitations exist in terms of potential range of movement?

   •   Work through the joints of the body relating the type of joint to the movement potential.

2   Analyse the major muscle groups involved in a specific movement in your sport. Identify the prime mover, antagonist and stabiliser muscle (s) and the type of muscle action involved. Identify the types of muscle fibre used and why they are suited to that role.

CHAPTER TWO:
How the Body Works

2.0 Introduction

To execute any activity (eg reading a book, walking to the shops) you need a continuous supply of energy. If exercise is to continue for any length of time, the delivery systems need to maintain the supply of energy to the working muscles. If insufficient, the body will slow down or stop the activity. A knowledge of the heart, lungs and circulatory system, together with their respective roles in energy production, is essential in understanding oxygen's contribution to the production of ATP (the energy *currency* of all the body's cells) and the physiological demands of sport.

The critical role that the circulation and lungs play in any sport can be clearly seen by observing a performer in action. The increase in rate and depth of breathing, along with the increase in temperature (reflected by reddening of the face), are obvious signs. Think about the end of any race or match and the appearance of the performers.

Less obvious is the increase in heart rate and blood lactate accumulation within the circulation. It is these less obvious effects of physical exertion that the coach must monitor carefully to appreciate fully the way in which muscles adapt so that effective training programmes can be developed to achieve maximum gains in performance.

2.1 Cardio-respiratory System

This system is responsible for transporting oxygen and food components (nutrients) to the working muscles and removing metabolites involved in energy conversion and respiration (eg lactate and carbon dioxide). The cardio-respiratory system consists of the lungs and associated airways, the heart, blood and blood vessels (Figure 28 page 39).

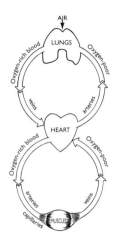

Figure 28: Flowchart of the cardio-respiratory system

Airways

Air is breathed in through the nose and mouth, where it is warmed and filtered en route to the back of the throat (**pharynx**). It then passes through the voice-box (**larynx**) which contains the epiglottis, a flap which prevents food entering the windpipe (**trachea**). The trachea forms a single airway which divides into the left and right bronchi. These subdivide to smaller and smaller branches (**bronchioles**) which carry air to the air sacs (**alveoli**) lining the lungs (page 45). In each lung there are about 150 million alveoli with a total surface area equivalent to a tennis court. Oxygen diffuses from the alveoli across the walls of the network of blood capillaries and into the red blood cells. At the same time, carbon dioxide moves in the opposite direction, from the blood into

the alveoli, to be carried back to the bronchioles and eventually exhaled. During exercise the blood flowing through the capillaries speeds up, taking about 0.25 seconds to pass over an alveolus. This matches the time taken for oxygen to pass from the air in the alveolus to the blood.

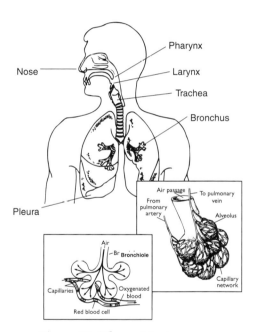

Figure 29: The respiratory system

Breathing

The lungs are made of elastic tissue which is unable to contract. They change in volume as a result of pressure changes between the inside and outside of the lungs due to the changing shape of the chest (thoracic cavity). As the thorax expands, the volume in the lungs increases, the pressure drops and air is drawn into the lungs (page 45) by flowing down the pressure gradient (ie from relatively higher pressure outside to the alveoli, where the pressure is relatively lower). To breathe out, the muscles of the diaphragm relax, the thorax returns to its original size, pressure increases in the lungs forcing air out. The diaphragm, which is at the base of the thoracic cavity, divides the thorax from the abdomen.

Muscular contraction flattens the diaphragm causing the volume of the thorax to increase. This reduces the internal pressure relative to the outside and air flows in. As the diaphragm flattens, the pressure in the abdominal cavity increases causing the stomach wall to move out, even at rest. Respiration rate at rest is controlled by the changes in carbon dioxide concentration in the blood rather than the need for oxygen. During exercise, breathing rate is probably increased by the combination of an increase in nerve activity originating in the chest wall and factors in the blood (eg increased carbon dioxide and decreased oxygen).

The importance of the pressure difference is illustrated in the case of a punctured lung. If a hole exists between the outer body and the thorax (or the thorax and the lungs), it is impossible to create a pressure difference and so change the shape of the lungs. If the lungs cannot enlarge or shrink, air does not pass in or out of the lungs, and so oxygen cannot diffuse into the blood.

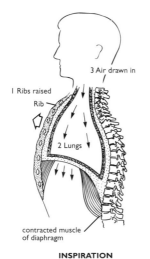

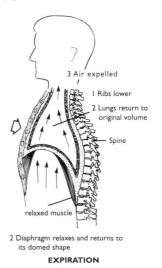

Figure 30: Movements involved in breathing

TASK

The following test can be used to show the effect of carbon dioxide on breathing rate:

1 Time how long you can hold your breath.

2 Breathe in and out deeply 10–15 times.

3 Now time how long you can hold your breath.

The reason you can hold your breath longer the second time is due to the forced expellation of carbon dioxide from the lungs. The more efficient the lungs become at removing the build up of carbon dioxide, the greater the oxygen supply available to fuel the muscles during periods of intense aerobic activity. Notice how your breathing rate changes during exercise. Does it become faster or slower with training?

Heart

The heart (Figure 31) is a muscle which acts as a dual action, or suction, pump, continually circulating blood throughout the body. The right side of the heart is completely separate from the left. Each consists of two chambers, a ventricle and an atrium.

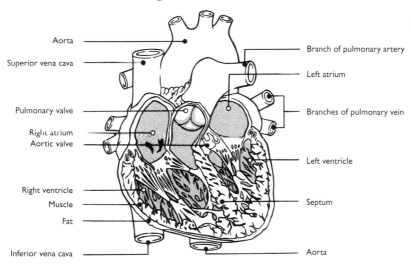

Figure 31: The heart

The atria carry out the following functions:

- The **left atrium** receives oxygenated blood from the lungs via the pulmonary vein and passes it to the left ventricle.

- The **left ventricle** pumps the oxygenated blood into the aorta (major artery from the heart) and into the arteries, arterioles and capillaries throughout the body.

- The **right atrium** receives deoxygenated (reduced oxygen) blood via the superior and inferior vena cava (major veins to the heart) from the capillaries, venules and veins from the rest of the body. Blood passes from the right atrium to the right ventricle.

- The **right ventricle** pumps the deoxygenated blood into the pulmonary artery which transports blood to the lungs where carbon dioxide is expelled and oxygen absorbed.

Although the two sides contract simultaneously, they form two separate circulatory systems:

- **Systemic** circulation (to and from the rest of the body).
- **Pulmonary** circulation (to and from the lungs).

The aortic valve separates the aorta from the left ventricle preventing blood flowing back into the ventricle, allowing adequate pressure to build up for the efficient pumping of blood into the systemic circulation. The pulmonary valve separates the pulmonary artery from the right ventricle preventing blood flowing back into the right ventricle. At rest, the heart pumps about five litres of blood per minute. In a highly trained performer, this output can rise to 30 litres or more during exercise.

The systolic blood pressure reading represents the pressure when the heart is contracting and the diastolic blood pressure when it is relaxed (ie the beating action of the heart).

In a highly fit individual, readings will be lower than for the less fit due to the effects of training which are explained later in this chapter.

The normal range of blood pressure for relatively healthy individuals is 120–140 mmHg systolic and 60–90 mmHg diastolic. This varies with age, sex and *fitness* level, and is elevated by stress.

Blood Vessels

Collectively, the **blood vessels** are known as the vascular system. This consists of the following:

- **Arteries** transport oxygenated blood away from the heart to the muscles or organs. One exception is the pulmonary artery which transports deoxygenated blood to the lungs from the heart. Arteries are characterised by a narrow internal diameter (**lumen**) lined with smooth involuntary muscle.

- **Veins** transport deoxygenated blood from the muscles or organs to the heart. One exception is the pulmonary vein which transports oxygenated blood from the lungs to the heart. Veins are characterised by a large internal diameter (**lumen**) and, apart from the vena cava, all have valves to prevent a backflow of blood.

- **Capillaries** are the minute blood vessels where all the exchanges occur. Here the muscle fuels (eg blood glucose and free fatty acids – Chapter Three page 59) diffuse out of the capillaries to the muscle, accompanied by oxygen. At the same time carbon dioxide diffuses in the opposite direction, from the muscle to the capillaries.

During physical exertion, the work load of the blood vessels increases to ensure adequate transport of nutrients and oxygen to the muscles, as well as the removal of metabolites and carbon dioxide.

TASK

A rower relies on the rapid and effective transport of oxygen-rich blood by the arteries to supply the working muscles of the arms and legs to maintain rhythm and speed of the stroke. At the muscle site the capillaries supply the muscle with oxygen. The larger the surface area of the capillaries, the greater the advantage to the performer. As the muscles begin to work at increased intensity (eg interval training, sprints) metabolites of exercise (eg lactate) begin to accumulate. The contraction of large muscle groups will assist the return of the carbon dioxide-rich blood through the veins to the heart and lungs.

Analyse the way in which your sport will use this system and the significance of each of the blood vessels in maintaining activity.

Blood

The average man has about five litres of blood circulating in his body, women have about 10% less. Of greatest interest to performers is the ability of the circulatory system (blood transports oxygen and nutrients) to transport oxygen to the muscles and then take away metabolites and metabolic intermediaries, such as carbon dioxide and lactate.

Blood contains the following components:

- **Plasma**, which is a fluid containing the blood cells and transports proteins, salts, ions, oxygen, carbon dioxide, enzymes, lactate and hormones.

- Red blood cells (**erythrocytes**) which make up more than 99% of the blood cells. Their function is to transport oxygen in the chemical compound haemoglobin, which has a high affinity for oxygen.

- White blood cells (**leukocytes**) which protect against infection.

- **Platelets** which assist in blood clotting.

A healthy person at rest carries around 200ml of oxygen in each litre of arterial blood (one-fifth of its volume). A litre of venous blood, which has given up oxygen to the muscles during exercise, may hold as little as 30ml of oxygen per litre. Obviously, it is necessary for the blood to contain enough haemoglobin if the muscles are to work efficiently. The haemoglobin content is measured in grams per 100ml of blood, and again there is a slight difference between men and women. Men will have between 14–16g per 100ml, and women about 12–14g. If the haemoglobin content drops below these figures, anaemia is said to exist.

Lactate is generated as a metabolic intermediary of the anaerobic energy system – specifically anaerobic glycolysis (Section 3.10 page 87). It is eventually removed from the blood in various ways:

- Lactate can be removed and neutralised as a metabolic fuel mostly by cardiac muscle and, to a degree, by skeletal muscle.

- Some of the protons are dissociated and turned into carbon dioxide which is later exhaled.

- Some is cleared by the action of the heart muscle, brain, liver and kidney tissues.

Refer to Chapter Three page 59 for details on energy conversion.

Low haemoglobin (Hb) levels mean less oxygen is available to the working muscles which can ultimately lead to reduced endurance. Hb contains iron, therefore low iron intakes or excessive losses can lead to anaemia. Female performers tend to be more susceptible to anaemia due to losses through menstruation.

Coaches and performers should be aware of the symptoms of anaemia: possible flu-like symptoms with accompanying mood changes such as depression and a possible reduction in performance. The practice of compensating with excessive iron supplements can have adverse effects (eg diarrhoea, abdominal pain and constipation) and should be carefully monitored. A sports dietitian or sports doctor should be consulted to diagnose and treat anaemia.

2.2 Lungs at Work

At rest, about ten litres of air is breathed in per minute. During really hard exercise, this can readily go up to 120 litres and sometimes 150 litres or higher (up to 200 litres in extreme cases). About 50 litres per minute is the maximum that can be breathed in through the nose; after that, breathing through the mouth is necessary. During mouth breathing, the air is not warmed or moistened as much as normal, so if a performer exercises unusually hard on a particularly cold or dry day, a slight burning pain may be felt afterwards in the midline of the chest, just below the breastbone. This is nothing to worry about; it simply indicates a slight inflammation of the mucous membrane lining the trachea or windpipe.

It is more efficient for performers to take fewer, larger breaths than many small ones. The breathing rates of female squash players have been observed to rise above 50 breaths per minute when doing intensive shadow training on the court. Strangely enough, even with extensive endurance training (Section 4.2 page 99), very little happens to the lungs. Their capacity does increase due to greater elasticity of the air sacs and stronger respiratory muscles. The volume of air moved in and out of the lungs at rest is much the same before and after training but there is a marked improvement in the maximum volume that can be moved during exercise. What actually improves is not getting the oxygen in but transporting it away, which is the job of the heart.

2.3 Heart at Work

The amount of blood pumped by the heart per minute is known as the **cardiac output**. The cardiac output will increase in proportion to the intensity of exercise. It does so by the following:

- An increase in the amount of blood pumped by the left ventricle in one single beat (**stroke volume**). This may increase from a resting level of around 85ml to an exercise level of 130ml in adults (stroke volumes of up to 210ml per beat have been seen in Olympic medal winning cross-country skiers).

- The **heart rate**, which will increase from resting values to maximum rates according to the intensity of the exercise. The maximum rate decreases with age. A very rough, approximate, maximum heart rate can be found by subtracting the person's age from 220 (eg a 20 year old should have a maximum heart rate of about 200 beats per minute; 220–20=200). The maximum heart rate is the same for both sexes. On average, the hearts of males are about 10% larger and heavier than females, even when total body weight measurements are taken into account.

Coaches must be aware that calculating the maximum heart rate by subtracting age from 220 is not totally accurate and should be used only as a rough guideline. Differences of 10% either way can occur depending on the individual's characteristics.

Training Effect on the Heart

With exercise and training, the heart adapts to meet the new demands in a number of ways:

- **Size.** The heart is a muscle and will therefore respond to training by increasing in size. Most notable differences are evident in the left ventricle which pumps out blood to the rest of the body. Road cyclists and rowers generally have the largest hearts in relation to their body weight.

- **Stroke volume.** The increase in heart size and strength enables an increase in chamber volume allowing more blood to be pumped per beat.

- **Resting heart rate.** As the heart becomes more efficient, the demands during both exercise and rest can be met with less effort. The heart rate will decrease (**bradycardia**) as it is able to pump much larger volumes per beat. In extreme cases the resting pulse may drop below 40 beats per minute (eg Miguel Indurain, five times winner of the *Tour de France* – 29 bpm). Average readings for performers range from 55–70 bpm depending on fitness levels. Submaximal exercising heart rate will decrease as the condition (*fitness*) of the performer improves.

- **Cardiac output** (the volume of blood pumped by the heart per unit of time, usually one minute). It is the product of the heart rate (rate at which the heart beats) and stroke volume (amount of blood pumped per beat). Training improvements lead to an overall increase in total cardiac output.

- **Blood volume and haemoglobin.** Both the total blood volume and the total amount of haemoglobin increase with training.

Limiting Factors

With training the bigger, stronger heart increases its output of blood. However, at very high heart rates (eg 90–95% of maximum), the heart's problem is in filling its chambers, not emptying them. Over two-thirds of the time from one beat to the next is occupied by the heart filling up again. With a heart rate of 180 beats per minute, there is only one-third of a second for a complete heart cycle, which means that about one-fifth of a

TASK

The release of the hormone *adrenaline* (one of the *catecholamines*) contributes to the redistribution of blood to the working muscles during physical activity. It also helps to increase heart rate, raises blood pressure and mobilises fatty acid and glucose in the blood for energy. A relatively small, anticipatory rise of adrenaline occurs just before the start of exercise. However, a larger, sudden release can occur in response to a sudden fright or shock – this is often referred to as the *flight or fight response*.

Think about a situation when you have become excited before a sporting or non-sporting event (eg prior to an academic examination). Try to remember how you felt (eg nervous stomach, heart beating faster) shortly before that event.

second is available for refilling and this is just about the minimum time needed. The heart muscle (**myocardium**) itself receives a blood flow during the relaxation and filling period (**diastole**). If the maximum heart rate is too high, there is not enough time for a good blood flow to, and oxygenation of, the myocardium. The filling problem of the heart has another implication when performers stop very strenuous activity suddenly (as in stopping immediately at the end of a 1500 metre race, or coming straight off a squash court and standing still at the conclusion of a long hard rally). They may feel quite giddy or possibly faint.

This condition occurs because during exercise, the heart is pumping out around 25 litres of blood a minute, and the muscles are delivering 25 litres a minute back to the heart by progressively squeezing the blood up the one-way veins, aided by the breathing movements of the chest. If exercise stops very suddenly, then the heart goes on pumping blood out but the return of venous blood is suddenly cut down as blood pools in the limbs. The heart cannot pump out what it does not receive, so the blood pressure drops rapidly and the performer may feel faint. This is not at all serious but does indicate the need to cool-down for at least two minutes after the event has stopped.

It is also important that the heart should not be overloaded in training or competition. If the performer is or

Even allowing for body size, **children** can only supply a fraction of the oxygen requirements of working muscles, compared with adolescents and adults. Children breathe faster and less deeply than adults during exercise and they are not able to extract as much oxygen from the air:

- They must work harder to gain the required amount of oxygen to the muscles.

- Breathing hard increases the rate at which the body loses water and they are, therefore, more susceptible to dehydration.

- Coaches must ensure that young performers do not overwork and drink small quantities frequently.

has suffered from any illness associated with raised body temperature, particularly a viral condition, it is possible that the virus has infiltrated the heart muscle leading to inflammation. If the muscles still feel sore due to a viral infection, the heart rate should not be raised by training – performers should be forced to rest. The dangers are very real and have proved fatal. For this reason, it is important that performers do not exercise hard with an upper respiratory tract infection (a cold) which is in the chest.

Fitness and Heart Disease

With increasing fitness, the number of capillary blood vessels within the muscles also increases. In certain areas this can be by as much as 50%. As a heart attack (coronary thrombosis) is a blockage of the coronary artery, any increase in the number of capillaries of the heart tends to limit the extent of muscle damage within the heart as the result of a heart attack. It is the size of the affected area that often makes the critical difference between life and death, so training could eventually contribute to survival.

Measuring Heart Rate

Coaches and performers should monitor heart rate as accurately as possible, as this can provide a good indication of training intensity and recovery. The pulse itself is a shock wave produced by the blood surging out of the heart at each beat as it travels along the arteries. The pulse may be easy to locate if it is very distinct but in most individuals it can often be quite difficult to locate quickly. The best places to locate the pulse are at the wrist (**radial** pulse) and in the neck (**carotid** pulse). To locate the radial pulse (Figure 32), it may be necessary to press quite hard at the base of the thumb (care must be taken not to press too hard as this will stop the pulse and you will not be able to feel it).

To find the carotid pulse, the neck must only be pressed lightly. If it is pressed too hard, it may reduce the blood supply to the brain and cause feelings of dizziness. There is a natural reflex which slows the heart if the carotid artery is squeezed, which will give a false indication of heart rate. The pulse should be located with the fingers rather than the thumb as the thumb has its own distinct pulse.

The use of heart rate training zones allows for the differences in age but not gender of an individual. Heart rate monitors are commercially available and offer an effective and convenient guide to training intensities.

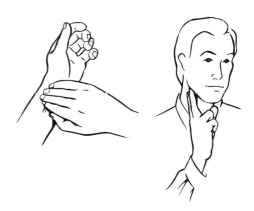

Figure 32: Locating the pulse

Yvonne Murray (Olympic 3000 metre medal winner in the 1992 Barcelona Games) adapts her training sessions according to her morning pulse count. If it is 4–5 beats higher than normal, she will avoid high intensity training that day to allow her body adequate time to recover fully.

Think how pulse rate monitoring can assist the coach in maximising performance and protecting against fatigue and overtraining. Is it used in your sport?

2.4 Factors Affecting Blood

There is only a limited amount of blood within the circulatory (or vascular) system. During exercise the body re-routes the blood to the working muscles where it is needed most and reduces the amount flowing in other areas (eg to the liver and kidneys). The body does this by increasing the diameter of the arteries supplying blood to the working muscles (vasodilation) and by decreasing the diameter of the arteries in other parts of the body, which are not directly involved in the activity (vasconstriction).

Normally at rest, about 40% of the entire output of the heart goes to the liver and kidneys. With the onset of vascular redistribution, it is markedly reduced from 40% to about 5%. Similarly blood is directed away from the abdominal and pelvic organs (eg stomach and intestines and also from the skin). It is this movement away from the skin that makes some performers look rather pale just before their event or match.

This redistribution away from the liver in those who are not very highly trained is almost certainly one cause of a stitch, particularly the stitch that is felt at the right shoulder (some liver pain is felt here, just as some heart pain is felt in the left arm). The sudden reduction of blood in the liver causes it to shrink in size, which strains the stretch receptors in its covering membrane, producing the pain.

This may also be one cause of the butterflies felt in the abdomen just before a competition. However, the net result is that some 30% of the cardiac output becomes newly available for circulation to the muscles.

TASK

It is important for coaches and performers to understand the consequences of blood distribution, particularly during periods of increased intensity. Circulation problems might occur when a performer needs an increase in blood supply to the working muscles (eg a gymnast performing a series of continuous tumbles and jumps) but this increase in activity coupled with the room temperature will create heat energy.

To maintain a constant body temperature, blood flow to the skin needs to increase to release this excess heat by radiation. If the muscles continue to demand oxygen the performer is faced with the possibility of overheating, particularly in the case of endurance runners where the large leg muscles demand heavy increases in blood flow to sustain performance.

Think about the possible implications in your sport and preventative measures that can be taken (eg wearing the appropriate clothing for warm-up and cool-down periods, limiting the amount of clothing during intense activity, increasing fluid intake).

Anaemia

Anaemia is a condition of the blood in which the number of functional red blood cells or their haemoglobin content is below normal. It can result from a decrease in the:

- number of red blood cells (erythrocytes)

- amount of haemoglobin in each erythrocyte or a combination of the two.

When training performers for aerobic endurance, the important measure is the amount of oxygen-carrying haemoglobin. As already mentioned, the amount of haemoglobin in healthy men is between 14–16g per 100ml of blood; in women between 12–14g. If the haemoglobin content is much less than these figures, a greater or lesser degree of anaemia may be said to be present. Cases of anaemia do occur, especially in young women who have prolonged periods of menstruation. However, a considerable number of aerobic endurance performers of either sex might be diagnosed as having clinical anaemia when they have what could be more accurately termed sports anaemia. This is because one of the results of aerobic endurance training is an overall increase in the amount of blood in the body.

Hypervolaemia may involve increases of up to 50% but curiously enough the red cell increase does not quite match the plasma (fluid) increase, so although there is much more blood and therefore more haemoglobin in total, the actual concentration of red cells is less. Thus aerobic endurance performers may well be at the bottom of (or even below) the normal haemoglobin range, purely as a natural response to training.

March Haemoglobinurea

This is a condition (first observed in marching soldiers) which mainly affects long-distance runners. About 5% of distance runners (usually men) notice that their urine is discoloured after a long run on the road; it may be brownish or slightly reddish and naturally enough this can give rise to some anxiety. However, this symptom is simply due to the way the capillaries in the soles of the feet react to sustained pounding. This releases some haemoglobin, which circulates in the blood and then slips through the kidney filters, eventually appearing in the urine. The effect seems to be quite harmless although medical consultation must be sought to confirm diagnosis and ensure there are no serious complications.

Altitude Effect

Exposure to altitudes higher than 1500–2500m (usually referred to as *moderate altitude*) for 2–3 weeks is believed to stimulate an increase in red cell production (**polycythemia**) to counteract the *thinner* air. This may lead to a greater concentration of red blood cells in the blood (ie haemoglobin content) and may result in an increased oxygen carrying capacity. There is still much controversy and disagreement about altitude training.

An increase in red blood cell concentration makes the blood thicker; it becomes more viscous and therefore harder for the heart to pump. As the red blood cell count increases, the maximum heart rate reduces. During the early stages of altitude exposure, submaximal exercise heart rate and cardiac output may increase by up to 50% above sea level values, whereas the heart's stroke volume remains unchanged. It could be more beneficial for performers to have short duration (no more than three weeks) stays at altitude to improve performance.

Altitude acclimatisation is essential if a performer is going to compete at altitude; the length of acclimatisation period depends on the altitude at which the performer will compete. Acclimatisation at one altitude ensures only partial adjustment to a higher elevation. As a broad guideline, approximately two weeks are required to adapt to altitudes up to 2300m. Thereafter, for every 610m increase, an additional week is necessary to adapt fully up to an altitude of approximately 4600m. In addition, because central limitations (ie cardiorespiratory) occur first, the muscles begin to decondition.

Research on training at altitude remains inconclusive as to whether such methods provide any additional benefits to sea-level performance, compared with equivalent training at sea level. This seems to be due to the various reductions in physiological function, in that both maximum heart rate and stroke volume are reduced.

Blood Doping

Blood doping is an illegal way of reproducing the benefits of a stay at altitude (increased red blood cell concentration). A certain volume of blood is removed from the performer, whose body will generally replenish the loss within a week. The blood is stored and some weeks later, the same blood is transfused back again. This procedure does increase aerobic endurance but its timing can be difficult, the results are not always predictable and it may lead to a drop in natural red blood cell production some weeks later.

More recently some performers have started using synthetically manufactured **erythropoetin** (EPO) which provides the same effect as altitude training and blood doping. It too is illegal but difficult to detect.

Sweating and Body Fluids

Sweating is part of the body's heat-regulating mechanism – cooling the skin, during exposure to heat, by evaporation. In order for the sweat to evaporate from the surface of the skin, it requires energy which it obtained from the heat of the skin warmed by the blood. The amount of fluid lost as sweat is considerable; for example squash players, marathon runners and footballers can lose over two litres per hour.

Training affects the sweat pattern of performers. Trained people generally begin sweating sooner than the untrained. The sweat produced by trained athletes is far more dilute, containing approximately half the usual concentration of salts (eg sodium, potassium and magnesium chlorides).

Sweating reduces total blood volume resulting in dehydration. During vigorous exercise, fluid is shifted from the blood. One result of this is to increase the concentration of red cells.

However, when sweating starts in earnest, the sweat glands derive the water directly from the blood. If performers sweat more than half their blood volume during competition, the body compensates by taking advantage of its three fluid reserves:

- The blood itself.
- The interstitial fluid which is between all body cells.
- The fluid inside all body cells.

There is a reserve of three times the blood plasma volume held between the cells and a further ten times that volume inside the cells. These reservoirs keep the blood topped up as it loses fluid to the sweat glands. As these reserves are used up, dehydration begins to occur. Dehydration leads to increased body temperature and lowered output of the heart resulting in decreases in performance.

The adequate replacement of sweat loss is vital in maintaining performance and preventing disorders such as heat stroke and heat exhaustion. Thirst is not a good indication of fluid loss as only after 2% of body weight has been lost, does a performer feel thirsty. Losing 2% of body weight as fluid can lead to a 20% decrease in performance. In extreme conditions (eg exercise), it is essential to consume frequent small amounts of fluid before, during and after exercise. It is not possible to replace all the lost fluid in this way as during exercise, blood flow to the intestine is reduced and therefore less water can be absorbed. When the exercise is over, this remaining fluid debt is progressively repaid. At this stage it is also important to replace the lost salts.

There is also an increased risk of dehydration from sweat loss when exercising in cold environments (eg ice hockey players wear a lot of clothing and equipment; consequently they lose a lot of body fluid through sweating).

As much as 60% of a performer's body weight is water, a loss of one and a half litres could cause dehydration to many individuals and seriously impair performance. A marathon runner on a hot day could quite easily lose this amount in as little as 30 minutes. You can monitor fluid loss by regularly weighing yourself before and after training sessions. Simply remember that one kilogramme of body weight is equal to one litre of fluid. However, for each kilogramme lost, a performer should drink one and a half litres of fluid, as a third is immediately converted to urine.

While the same physiological principles apply to children as to adults, coaches should be aware that children adapt, respond and cope differently.

- Children have a relatively large surface area to volume ratio compared with adults and tend to exchange heat faster:

  - They tend to overheat more easily in hot weather.

  - In cold weather they lose heat more quickly and become cold

  - Coaches must carefully monitor young performers for any adverse signs during exercise in hot or cold environments.

- Children tend to overheat in hot environments:

  - They should be encouraged to drink small quantities frequently and need to drink before, during and after activity (especially in warm weather).

  - They should never feel thirsty or dry in the mouth.

  - Remember to discourage performers of all ages and standards from sharing drinking bottles to prevent germs from being transmitted.

- Children require adequate rest during and between training sessions or competition:

  - Coaches must plan and organise training or competition to allow for adequate recovery.

  - Adequate recovery will prevent staleness, promote enjoyment and adaptation to training.

Coaches must be highly observant during all activities and pay particular attention to the individual needs of their performers.

2.5 Factors Affecting Lung Function

The more common conditions and situations which can affect lung function are listed below:

- Asthma
- Bronchitis, due to irritants (eg cigarette smoking, air pollution, infection)
- Cystic fibrosis
- Lung cancer (really only significant in smokers).

Asthma

Asthma is an increasingly common disease where the respiratory airways constrict, reducing the rate of airflow to the lungs making breathing (particularly exhalation) difficult. The added danger is that oxygenation of the blood will be reduced. It can be caused by a number of factors including allergy, pollution, stress, infection and in some cases, exercise.

Approximately 5% of the population are asthma sufferers and with continuing amounts of pollutants in the atmosphere, these numbers are set to increase further. The pollen, dust or smoke acts by irritating the lining of the airways causing inflammation or swelling and resulting in the individual struggling for breath.

Some individuals exhibit asthmatic symptoms only when they exercise (ie exercise induced asthma). This is believed to be caused by the cooling and drying of the airways which can occur after exercise in certain conditions. Post-exercise airway constriction is perhaps a better name for the condition, since the effects are not fully evident until about 15 minutes after exercise. Exercise induced asthma seems to occur much less in swimming, where there is a warm and moist environment, than in running.

Asthma can often be controlled by medication (eg Intal, Ventolin and Bricanyl), so most competing asthmatics can continue in their sport. Intal, taken about 30 minutes before the exercise, is very useful in preventing attacks from occurring; Ventolin and Bricanyl are effective in controlling an attack. Asthma sufferers should always discuss doping control regulations with team medical officers.

If an asthmatic performer gets into difficulty during activity and an inhaler is not at hand, the coach or performer must improvise. It is possible to inflate a small paper or plastic bag with air so the performer can inhale the air into the lungs. Coaches and performers should avoid group use or the borrowing of other people's inhalers as this could both infringe doping control regulations and transmit germs and/or disease. If a performer does have an attack, all activity should stop.

Asthmatics who have a respiratory tract infection should try to avoid any physical activity. Allergic asthma sufferers should try to avoid allergic substances/environments, and should take various steps towards reducing the risk of allergic attacks (eg regular cleaning or vacuuming of bedroom or working environment).

2.6 Summary

To recognise fully how the body moves in sporting situations, it is essential to understand the physical changes that occur within the body to provide the energy for movement. A knowledge of the systems responsible for supplying the oxygen and nutrients to the working muscles and the pathways used to remove waste products, is fundamental to achieving maximum gains. This knowledge will be of significant benefit when devising effective and safe training programmes and optimising performance in competition.

Further detailed information can be found in the following reference books:

Berne, P and Levy, S (1996) **Principles of physiology**. London, Mosby. ISBN 0 815105 23 1

Clegg, C (1995) **Exercise physiology and functional anatomy**. New Milton, Feltham Press. ISBN 0 9520743 1 1

*Farrally, M (1991) **An introduction to sports physiology**. Leeds, National Coaching Foundation and Scottish Sports Council (Home Study Pack). ISBN 0 947850 96 1

Available from **Coachwise 1st4sport** (tel 0113-201 5555 or visit www.1st4sport.com).

Fox, E and Bowers, R (1998) **The physiological basis for exercise and sport.** London, McGraw-Hill Education. ISBN 0 071158 99 5

Lamb, J and Ingram, C (1991) **The essentials of physiology.** 3rd edition, Oxford, Blackwell Scientific. ISBN 0 632 03135 2

Reilly, T and Secher, N (1990) **Physiology of sports.** London, E & F N Spon. ISBN 0 419 13590 1

Wilmore, J and Costill, D (1999) **Physiology of sport and exercise.** Champaign IL, Human Kinetics. ISBN 0 736000 84 4

TASK

The following task will help you test your understanding of the oxygen transport system and how it supplies the working muscles with the required fuel for your sport.

During a training session, record the pulse rate at the following intervals:

1   At the start prior to activity.

2   After pulse raising exercises but before stretching.

3   After stretching.

4   After final pulse raising activity before main activity (if appropriate).

5   During and after main activity.

6   After cool-down activity (before stretching).

7   After final cool-down stretches.

Draw a graph with activity against pulse readings. How do the readings differ? Explain this in relation to the effects of exercise on the heart. Will all the participants' readings be the same? Explain your findings.

CHAPTER THREE:
Nutrition and the Energy Systems

3.0 Introduction

Movement is fuelled by energy provided from the breakdown of food and drink. A well-balanced diet will ensure performers maximise and maintain the training programme needed to achieve their ultimate potential in competition. Coaches need to understand basic nutritional principles as well as how the energy systems work within the body.

An individual's potential will depend on both uncontrollable factors (eg genetics, age, gender and body type) and controllable factors (eg training effects and nutrition). Nutrition will be described in this chapter through the identification of the nutrients required for normal functioning of the body and sports performance.

Good nutritional sources will be discussed as well as the overall effect of a well balanced, energy dense diet on performance. The energy systems will be described by breaking down the various systems into their individual components.

3.1 Why Food is Needed

Food is essential for a number of reasons:

- **Energy.** Every living cell in the body requires energy to function adequately in order to maintain the natural balance of the body **(homeostasis).**

- **Growth and repair of tissue.** To promote growth, repair and strengthening of muscle, bone, tendons and ligaments.

- **General body functioning.** Nutrients are required by the body for many essential processes including tissue regeneration, oxygen transportation and the functioning of the digestive tract.

3.2 Principles of Nutrition

The principles of nutrition initially can seem complex and diverse but can be simplified by viewing the components in a systematic way. The terms and components will be defined and explained more fully.

Diet

Diet refers to a particular pattern of eating and drinking habits. A well-balanced diet will provide adequate amounts of protein, vitamins, minerals and energy required for tissue maintenance, repair, growth and energy.

Nutrients

Food can be broken down into nutrients which are essential components of the diet. These include:

- Carbohydrates
- Fats
- Proteins
- Vitamins
- Minerals
- Water.

Carbohydrates, fats and proteins are the only sources of food energy; they are called the energy nutrients. Minerals and water are inorganic nutrients. Vitamins play an important role in every single cell of the body.

The energy trapped within the chemical bonds of carbohydrates, fats and proteins varies between foods and is converted during a series of complex chemical reactions to form **Adenosine Triphosphate** (ATP, the body's energy *currency* – Section 3.10 page 85).

Vitamins act as catalysts in normal metabolic processes of the body and minerals perform vital life functions (eg calcium plays an important role in the contraction and relaxation of skeletal muscle).

It is essential to consume a variety of foods, as no single food contains sufficient quantities of each nutrient to meet the demands of the body. Water is the most important nutrient required by the body and is vital in maintaining the many metabolic processes that sustain life.

It is not possible to state the specific amount of each nutrient needed by a given individual. The government has issued recommended intakes for certain nutrients as a guideline for assessing the adequacy of a population's nutrition. These values are termed **Dietary Reference Values** (DRV) and comprise the **Reference Nutrient Intake** (RNI) which indicates the requirement of each nutrient according to age, weight, lean body mass, growth, sex and level of activity. RNI represents the average so can only be used as a guideline by coaches and performers. Some individuals may have specific requirements of certain nutrients.

In this handbook the figures quoted for the recommended daily intake of specific nutrients have been taken from the government's COMA Report (1989). However, as part of the European Union's National Labelling directive (90/496/EEC) which came into effect on 1 March 1995, these reference values have been amended to reflect the differences between European countries and provide a standard for all food labelling.

This has had a significant effect on some of the values given on food packages and can affect energy calculations. For example the COMA Report (1989) suggested that the **Recommended Daily Allowance** (RDA) for Vitamin C is 30mg per day, where as the EEC RDA for Vitamin C is 60mg per day. The UK population recommended average is now 50% less than the EEC RDA. Coaches must be aware of the changes in terms of food labelling and energy content to ensure performers are achieving the RDAs based on proven scientific research.

Nutrition

This refers to the process by which chemicals from the environment are taken up by the body to provide the energy needed to keep the body alive, healthy and able to participate in physical activity.

Digestion

Digestion is the process by which the larger chemical compounds within foods are broken down by the digestive system into simple sugars, lipids and amino acids to be used by the body.

Absorption

This is the process where nutrients from the digested food, needed for energy conversion and bodily functions, move into the circulatory system from the stomach and small intestine. The blood transports the nutrients to where they are needed (eg muscle cells for contraction, body cells for growth and repair, and vital organs, fat cells for storage).

Excretion and Elimination

These terms refer to the removal of the metabolic wastes via the kidney (eg urine) and the removal of the nondigestible material from the digestive process, residues of digestive juices from the intestines, stomach and pancreas, and old, broken-down red blood cells, bacteria and foreign particles (eg faeces).

3.3 Energy

Almost every function performed by cells in the body requires energy. The nutrients consumed in the daily diet provide the necessary energy to generate ATP to maintain bodily functions both at rest and during physical activity.

The energy within food is measured in terms of the amount of heat that would be liberated by its complete breakdown in the body. Both energy expended and energy consumed is measured in either kilocalories (Kcal) or kilojoules (Kj).

The energy in the diet is mainly obtained from carbohydrates, fats and proteins (minimal amount). Although vitamins and minerals do not yield energy, they are essential for proper bodily function. The energy density differs considerably between nutrients. When fully oxidised, the energy yields are as follows:

Carbohydrate	16Kj/4.0Kcal per gram
Protein	17Kj/4.0Kcal per gram
Fat	37Kj/9.0Kcal per gram
Alcohol	29Kj/7.0Kcal per gram

For example, one gram of carbohydrate will produce 16Kj of energy.

The daily amount of energy required is dependent on many factors (eg size, weight and exercise). The average daily energy expenditure is estimated to be 2700–2900 Kcal for men and 2000–2100 Kcal for women between the ages of 15–50 years.

Great variability exists, however, and this difference is largely determined by the individual's physical activity level. If more energy is consumed than is actually required, the excess will be stored as fat and weight will increase. Similarly, if the energy intake is not sufficient, the body's stores of fat and possibly muscle will be called upon to meet the demand and weight will be lost. The coach needs to ensure a suitable balance is achieved between energy expenditure and intake to maintain a performer's overall capacity to train and compete.

Basal metabolic rate (BMR) refers to the amount of energy an individual requires over 24 hours at rest (ie bed rest). As previously discussed, all body systems require energy even when the major muscles are not physically active. Women, on average, have a lower BMR than men because they are usually smaller, have more body fat and a lower percentage of muscle tissue. For a man and a woman of the same weight, the difference in BMR is around 150 kilocalories (per 24 hours). Even at rest, muscle requires more energy than fat.

On top of the energy associated with BMR, everyone has to carry out daily living activities such as washing, dressing, sitting and walking which increase the daily energy requirement. Any further physical activity, due to a strenuous job or taking part in exercise, requires more energy. The daily energy requirement for active individuals will therefore consist of three components:

Total daily energy needs = BMR + general living activity + exercise

Table 3: Average daily energy requirements (Mj) depending on individual and activity level

Age range in years	Occupational category	Energy requirement kcal	MJ
Girls			
9 to 12		2300	9.6
12 to 15		2300	9.6
15 to 18		2300	9.6
Women			
18 to 55	most occupations	2200	9.2
	very active	2500	10.5
55 to 75	assumed sedentary	2050	8.6
75 and over		1900	8.0
During pregnancy (2nd and 3rd trimester)		2400	10.0
During lactation		2700	11.3
Boys			
9 to 12		2500	10.5
12 to 15		2800	11.7
15 to 18		3000	12.6
Men			
18 to 35	sedentary	2700	11.3
	moderately active	3000	12.6
	very active	3600	15.1
35 to 65	sedentary	2600	10.9
	moderately active	2900	12.1
	very active	3600	15.1
65 to 75	assumed sedentary	2350	9.8
75 and over		2100	8.8

TASK

A typical low-fat yoghurt contains various nutrients, which have differing energy yields:

Typical values	Per 100g	Approx per pot
Energy	323kj	405kj
Protein	3.9g	4.9g
Carbohydrate	13.5g	17.0g
(of which sugars)	13.5g	17.0g
Fat	1.1g	1.4g
(of which saturates)	0.9g	1.1g
Sodium	Trace	Trace
Fibre	Trace	Trace
Calcium	95mg	118mg (23% RDA)

Participation in sport generally requires a greater energy intake than normal daily activities. Look at the food wrappers and packages in your cupboard and try to list the amount of energy supplied. Which foods have the highest energy values in terms of kcal per gram and provide the greatest source of energy for the increased demands of your sport?

3.4 Nutrients

The primary concern of any performer's diet is the provision of adequate fuel to cope with the body's everyday requirements and to meet the extra energy requirements from training and competing. Most foods contain a combination of nutrients (carbohydrates, fats, proteins, vitamins, minerals and water) that all have specific roles to play.

Understanding the role of each will assist coaches and performers to devise effective dietary guidelines to maintain health and the capacity to train and compete.

Carbohydrates

The main function of carbohydrate is to serve as an energy fuel for the body. The energy derived from the breakdown of glucose (sugar) and glycogen is used to power muscular contraction as well as other normal body functions.

Carbohydrates are absorbed as sugars and then transported and moved to various sites of the body via the bloodstream. Carbohydrates will first enter the liver, move through the heart and then enter the bloodstream again.

The main types of carbohydrate are:

- **sugars:**

    - monosaccharides (eg glucose).

    - disaccharides (eg sucrose and maltose – sucrose is one molecule of glucose and one molecule of fructose joined together, maltose is two molecules of glucose joined together).

    - polymers (eg maltodextrins – chainlike structures of glucose joined together).

- **starches** (chainlike structures of glucose joined together).

A typical carbohydrate intake for a man in the UK is around 250–350g per day; a woman would consume around 150–300g each day. This should provide approximately 40–45% of total energy in the diet. The latest recommendations suggest more carbohydrate should be eaten, so that about a half (or possibly more) of the energy in a diet is provided by carbohydrate.

Glycaemic index

About 30 minutes after carbohydrate is eaten, blood glucose levels rise to a peak. This rise and subsequent fall of blood glucose level occurs at different rates depending on the type of food eaten and the person's rate of digestion. The glycaemic index (G-I) of a food is determined by the rate at which carbohydrate taken in the diet is available for digestion, absorption and glycogen resynthesis in the muscles. For the purpose of comparison, foods are compared to white bread (which has an arbitrary G-I of 100) in terms of their rate of carbohydrate digestion and muscle glycogen resynthesis. Therefore, foods containing carbohydrates can be classified according to the extent to which they increase the blood glucose concentration (eg high or low glycaemic index).

Foods with a high G-I (eg ice cream, white bread, chocolate) cause a rapid rise in blood glucose levels and those with a low G-I (eg rice, lentils, baked beans) tend to offer a more gradual and sustained rise in blood sugar.

The G-I only applies, however, to single foods. For example, if you eat bread with margarine or butter spread on it, the carbohydrate will not be as easily available to the body as it will take longer to be absorbed. The concept of the G-I of foods should be considered as a guideline only.

Timing of the food intake and its composition prior to and during competition is critical in optimising performance. A triathlete might seek a ready source of energy through the intake of simple carbohydrates (eg bar of chocolate). This can be absorbed very quickly into the bloodstream for instant energy conversion. However, if the concentration is too strong the body adapts to this rapid surge in the blood sugar level by secreting the hormone insulin which maintains and regulates blood sugar levels. In turn the performer's blood sugar level falls below normal due to this rise in insulin, which results in a lower than normal blood sugar level (hypoglycaemia). Instead of the triathlete increasing or sustaining intensity, performance can deteriorate as feelings of fatigue set in. If the initial energy source was based on a complex carbohydrate (eg bread roll), the gradual release of energy over time may contribute to the maintenance of blood sugar levels of the performer remaining constant, and possibly improve energy gains.

Select the foods which can best be consumed to meet the demands of your sport both before and during competition.

It is important to be aware that current research is still investigating the optimum sources of energy before and during activity and the relative concentrations.

Fats

Fats are also composed of carbon, hydrogen and oxygen although the proportion of oxygen is less than that in carbohydrate. Fats are important nutrients for the body, not only as a source of energy but also to synthesise many important compounds and tissues vital for normal functioning. They also provide an excellent carriage for fat-soluble vitamins (Vitamins A, D, E and K).

Although the potential energy source in fat is greater per gram than carbohydrates, a larger supply of oxygen and greater length of time is needed to break down the fat, making it less efficient. The basic component of a fat is the triglycerides (also known as *triacylglycerides*), which consists of a glycerol base with three fatty acids attached. The differences between the various types of fat depend upon which fatty acids are in the triglycerides. There are two main types:

- **Saturated fatty acids**, which are normally found in animal fats and are hard at room temperature (eg butter and lard).

- **Unsaturated fatty acids,** which are commonly found in vegetable or fish oils and are soft or liquid at room temperature. Two of these unsaturated fatty acids must be provided in the diet.

Contrary to popular belief, cholesterol is not a fatty acid but a type of fat found mainly in animal produce. When digested, triglycerides are broken down in the intestine to their constituent fatty acids and glycerol, which can then be absorbed. A typical fat intake is around 100–150g per day for men and 75–130g per day for women (approximately 40% or more of total energy intake).

However, the latest recommendations suggest the fat content of the diet should be reduced and provide no more than 35% of the total daily energy intake (a reduction of at least 12% of total fat intake for most individuals).

Proteins

Proteins are large molecules which the digestive system breaks down into simple units called amino acids. These contain carbon, hydrogen, oxygen, nitrogen and in some cases sulphur. There are 21 different amino acids but they can be combined together with enormous variety to create the different protein-based materials forming the body. There are eight which the body cannot produce for itself. These eight are known as essential amino acids and must be taken in as part of the diet.

Amino acids are required primarily for the manufacture of the structural components of many tissues such as

A typical quarter pounder (hamburger or beefburger) with cheese and fries will provide on average 729kcal of potential energy. Why then do a high percentage of top class performers avoid eating fast food to refuel energy stores? Think of the food wrappers you examined and the difference in the sources of total energy. A burger will certainly provide a lot of kcals but the fat content of 40g means that 52% of the total energy available comes from fat. Compare this with a jacket potato with chilli con carne which provides 340kcal per 100g; the relative fat contribution of 10.7g means only 29% of the total energy intake is derived from fat. As the body can use carbohydrate more efficiently in energy conversion, the lower the fat contribution, the greater the advantage to the performer. However, if the burger is adding to the total carbohydrate intake of a well balanced diet with the required levels of vitamins and minerals, then it will not adversely affect performance and will add variety to the diet.

muscle, haemoglobin, hormones and enzymes. Under certain circumstances (eg during periods of starvation or long endurance exercise), they may be used to provide energy.

When too much protein is consumed, the excess amino acids are broken down, the nitrogen excreted and the rest of the molecule converted and stored as fat. Deficiency of protein in the performer is rare – generally too much is consumed, usually in the form of animal protein. Research has indicated that during intense exercise, a small increase in protein intake is required. It must be stressed however, that this is a very individual concept and is relevant to other factors such as training intensity and recovery.

Foods containing high amounts of essential amino acids are meat, fish and dairy produce. However, the contribution made by non-animal sources (eg cereals, legumes, pulses and nuts) should not be overlooked. The traditional view of first class (animal) and second class (vegetable) proteins is not strictly true. It stems from the mistaken belief that the protein found in plants is of inferior quality. Vegetable proteins do contain essential amino acids but in smaller quantities. This deficiency can be overcome by eating plenty of different

types of vegetable protein. A typical protein intake is around 100g per day for a man and 75g per day for a woman. This provides approximately 10–15% of the total energy intake.

Vitamins are chemical compounds needed by the body in minute amounts to perform specific functions. In general they cannot be made by the body and so have to be consumed in the diet. Vitamins can be broadly classified into:

- **fat-soluble vitamins**
  (A, D, E and K)

- **water-soluble vitamins** (B and C).

In this country, obvious signs of vitamin deficiency in either the general public or the performer are rare. However, the possibility that low vitamin levels in the body may impair performance should not be overlooked.

Overconsumption of vitamins and minerals from food is rare but it is easy to consume 10–100 times more than is required by using concentrated vitamin and mineral supplements. Care should be taken, as the body cannot cope with non-physiological intakes of many vitamins (especially fat-soluble vitamins) without side effects. A summary of the role of the principal vitamins is given in Table 5.

Table 4: Recommended nutrient intake based on protein providing 14.7% of energy vitamins

	Protein g/d	Thiamin mg/d	Riboflavin mg/d	Niacin mg/d	B6 mg/d*	B12 mg/d	C mg/d	A mm/d
Males								
11–14 yrs	42.1	0.9	1.2	15	1.2	1.2	35	600
15–18 yrs	55.2	1.1	1.3	18	1.5	1.5	40	700
19–50 yrs	55.5	1.0	1.3	17	1.4	1.5	40	700
Females								
11–14 yrs	41.2	0.7	1.1	12	1.0	1.2	35	600
15–18 yrs	45.0	0.8	1.1	14	1.2	1.5	40	600
19–50 yrs	45.0	0.8	1.1	13	1.2	1.5	40	600

Table 5: Summary of sources and functions of vitamins

Vitamin		Sources	Involved in
A	Retinol or carotene	Liver, dairy produce, eggs, carrots, green leafy vegetables	Visual processes, connective tissue, skin
B1	Thiamin	Meat, whole grains, legumes, nuts	Carbohydrate metabolism CNS (central nervous system) function
B2	Riboflavin	Liver, dairy produce, meat, cereal;	Carbohydrate metabolism, vision, skin
B6	Pyridoxin	Meat, fish, green leafy vegetables, whole grains, legumes	Protein metabolism, red blood cell formation, CNS function
B12	Cyanocobalamin	Meat, fish, dairy produces – no vegetable sources	Red blood cell formation, CNS function
–	Niacin	Liver, meat, fish, peanuts, cereal products	Carbohydrate and fat metabolism
–	Folic acid	Liver, legumes, green leafy vegetables	Regulates growth of cells, including red blood cells
C	Ascorbic acid	Green leafy vegetables, fruit, potatoes, white bread	Connective tissue, iron absorption/metabolism, healing/infection
D	Calciferols	Dairy produce, action of sunlight on skin	Calcium metabolism, bones and teeth
E	Tocopherols	Vegetable oils, liver, green leafy vegetables, dairy produce, whole grains	Protects vitamins A & C, and fatty acids from destruction in body (anti-oxidant)
K		Green leafy vegetables and liver	Clotting of blood, fat digestion

TASK

Many performers and coaches consider taking vitamin supplements to enhance performance. Each individual will have different needs (eg a vegetarian endurance performer will have different needs from a non-vegetarian discus thrower). However, increases in exercise require an overall increase in food intake to provide the extra energy required. As long as the performer maintains a balanced diet appropriate to the demands of the sport, the vitamin intake should be adequate. It should be noted that excess water-soluble vitamins are passed out in the urine and excess fat-soluble vitamins are stored as fatty deposits in the body.

How might the use of vitamin supplements help certain performers in your sport? For example, an anaemic performer may need to take an iron supplement.

Minerals, Electrolytes and Trace Elements

Minerals are chemicals required by the body in very small amounts. They include iron, sodium, potassium, calcium, phosphorus and magnesium. They generally exist as mineral salts (eg sodium chloride) which when dissolved in water, separate into their constituent ions (sodium and chloride ions). Other chemicals (eg copper, zinc and fluoride) are required in extremely small quantities and are called trace elements.

They are all essential for life and are important components of bone, connective tissue, haemoglobin, hormones and many enzymes within the body. Excess consumption of some minerals, particularly when taken as supplements, can result in a toxic accumulation which may be harmful (eg iron by female performers).

Electrolytes, also known as mineral salts, break down into their constituent elements (eg sodium chloride splits to give sodium and chloride ions). They are present in most body fluids and assist in maintaining the electro-chemical gradient of many tissues, including muscle and nerve. Electrolytes are often included in commercial sports drinks (eg sodium chloride, potassium and magnesium) to replace those lost in sweat and help increase fluid absorption. For a summary of sources and functions of minerals, see page 71.

Table 6: Summary of sources and functions of minerals

Mineral	Sources	Involved in
Sodium	Salt, cheese, muscle/organ meat, fish/bacon	Neuromuscular transmission (nerve conduction) fluid and acid-base balance
Potassium	Meat, milk, vegetables, cereals, nuts	Neuromuscular transmission (nerve conduction) fluid and acid-base balance
Calcium	Milk, cheese, nuts, green vegetables, bread	Bone/tooth structure, nerve conduction, blood clotting
Magnesium	Green vegetables, meats, dairy produce, cereals	Neuromuscular transmission, bone formation, enzyme reactions - energy metabolism
Phosphorus	Grains and cereals, meat, milk, green vegetables	Bone/tooth formation, energy metabolism
Iro	Nuts/seeds, red muscle/organ meat, eggs, green vegetables	Haemoglobin/myoglobin formation
Zinc	Muscle meats, seafood, green vegetables	Enzyme synthesis
Copper	Shellfish, organ meats, nuts, legumes, cocoa/chocolate	Enzyme synthesis
Iodine	Seafood, eggs, dairy produce	Thyroid function
Fluoride	Seafood, water, tea	Tooth structure
Manganese	Nuts, dried fruit, cereals/grains, tea	Enzyme synthesis
Chromium	Meat, dairy products, eggs	Glucose/insulin metabolism
Selenium	Seafood, organ and muscle meats and grains	Anti-oxidant (membranes) election transfer

Some female performers who train at high intensity cease menstruating (athletic amenorrhea). This often coincides with a decrease in oestrogen production which can result in the onset of osteoporosis. Athletic amenorrhea may predispose female performers to early onset of this disorder. It has been found that the spinal bone mass is often lower in such performers. Female performers suffering from amenorrhea should consult a doctor to rule out any serious medical problems and should maintain an intake of 1500 milligrams of calcium per day. Weight gain, oestrogen replacement therapy and diet modification may be recommended by the doctor along with reduced training.

Fibre

As dietary fibre (roughage) is not actually absorbed by the body, it is often ignored. It is, however, an important part of the diet. Fibre is basically non-digestible material that forms the skeleton of plant cells. It is generally found on the outside of seeds, beans, peas and other vegetables. When outer layers of food are removed by milling or peeling, much of this important fibre is discarded. Fibre can be classified as insoluble or soluble.

Insoluble fibre (eg wheatbran) adds bulk to the gut contents, especially in the large intestine or colon where everything is absorbed. It speeds up the movement of the gut contents and makes passing faeces easier. A high fibre diet helps protect against cancer of the colon by promoting regular bowel movement. Faeces contain various cancer producing substances which can irritate the lining of the colon and cause cancer if left to accumulate. Unfortunately, wheat bran can also bind valuable minerals (eg iron, calcium, zinc) and prevent them from being absorbed, which explains why eating too much wheat bran can lead to mineral deficiency.

Soluble fibre (eg beans, lentils, oats, fruit) absorbs water to form a gel which adds bulk to the gut contents and dilutes potentially harmful toxins which are removed as faeces from the body.

The typical daily fibre intake of British men and women is about 15–25g. The latest recommendation is that increases in fibre intake to about 25–35g each day should be made. Exercise itself can be a powerful bowel stimulant, so the amount of fibre intake should be monitored to avoid frequent trips to the lavatory (particularly for endurance performers).

TASK

If you had to make just one change to your diet, changing from white to wholemeal bread would increase your fibre intake far more than eating more fruit and vegetables. What foods did you eat yesterday which were high in dietary fibre (eg cereals, fruit, pulses, root vegetables, leafy vegetables, nuts, seeds)?

How could you change this diet to increase the fibre content (eg change mid-morning snack of biscuits to eating a banana or dried fruit)?

Water

Water constitutes 40–60% of a person's body weight and is one of the most important substances required by the body. It performs numerous important functions:

- It is the main transportation mechanism in the body, at least by being the largest component of blood, conveying nutrients, waste materials and internal secretions (eg hormones) to target tissues.

- It is the prime component of many **cells** and as it is a powerful ionizing agent (a substance which increases the number of ions), it controls the distribution of numerous electrolytes within the cells and throughout the body (refer to minerals and trace elements). Similarly, oxygen and carbon dioxide as well as hydrogen ions which affect acidity changes, are dissolved in water.

- The role water plays in the regulation of the body's temperature is of vital importance, particularly during exercise. It performs this function by:

    - absorbing the heat generated during energy liberation and transporting it to the skin for eventual dissipation

    - excreting it as sweat which evaporates and has a cooling effect on the body.

It is important to note that even small losses of water (2–3% of body weight) can seriously impair performance. Performers must ensure they are always fully hydrated prior to exercise.

During exercise, fluid should be taken frequently but in small amounts, and performers should be encouraged to drink before they are thirsty. Rehydration must continue after exercise and should not be delayed. It is important that the body becomes conditioned to taking regular fluids to optimise performance.

Alcohol

Alcohol is the product of the fermentation of carbohydrate by yeasts. It may make a major contribution to a person's total energy intake. However, it differs from carbohydrate and fat in that it cannot be used by the muscles to provide energy during exercise. Furthermore, it cannot be used to provide a rapid release of energy on demand, as it is slowly metabolised by the liver at a constant rate.

Therefore, any energy derived from alcohol in excess of the energy requirement is simply stored as body fat. Additionally, excessive alcohol consumption can cause damage to the liver. Current recommended quantities of alcohol consumption indicate that four units per day for men and three units per day for women are unlikely to damage health (one unit = half pint of beer/lager, one glass of wine or a single measure of spirits). Current research suggests that one or two glasses of wine a day (particularly red), may lower the risks of heart disease.

3.5 Effects of Nutrition on Performance

The primary consideration for any performer is energy. People often fail to appreciate the way in which personal beliefs, likes and dislikes lead to eating habits which can seriously influence performance, both in training and competition. Eating habits greatly affect the provision of energy to the working muscles. It is only the carbohydrates, fats and proteins in food that can provide energy to the working muscles.

Carbohydrates and fats are the main fuels for the muscles; proteins are usually used when the supply of these is inadequate (eg if the performer is in a state of fasting or is undernourished). During most forms of exercise, the muscles principally derive energy from the stores of carbohydrate (as glycogen) within the muscles and the liver. The muscle derives energy from fat, mainly as free fatty acids, at the same time as burning carbohydrate. However, the muscle must use some carbohydrate to provide energy at a fast enough rate to match the speed at which it is being used during exercise. Even at relatively low exercise intensities, the rate at which energy can be converted by burning fats alone is not fast enough. Therefore, some of the limited glycogen reserves are always used every time exercise is taken and the body's reserves decrease during every training session.

It is the continual replenishment of these glycogen reserves between training sessions that is vital to ensure adequate fuel is available at future sessions. Without the necessary reserves, training intensity will decline because energy cannot be converted fast enough. Eventually, the level becomes so low that even the shortest session becomes difficult to complete, the quality of each session suffers and so does the performer. The refuelling capacity of the individual is primarily determined by diet and the coach must encourage the performer to replenish carbohydrate stores. Assistance may also be needed in organising an eating plan to coincide with training commitments so the performer will always be fully fuelled at the onset of each session, regardless of time of day.

Characteristics of puberty:

- Characterised by body growth, physical maturation and generally increased appetite.
- Muscle mass and fat deposition generally increase (in girls fat deposition can increase significantly).
- Psychological changes include altered nervous system and increased sexual drive.
- Coordinated growth of organs such as heart, liver, lungs and kidneys.

Nutritional demands of puberty:

- To fuel increased demands on the body an enhanced and balanced diet is essential to performers.
- Body growth and development not only require energy but also sufficient proteins, carbohydrates and essential fats to achieve sustained body growth.
- Performers need to balance the energy demands of growth and physical activity with energy intake.

Coaches must be aware of the following:

- Young performers are regularly monitored and given sufficient time to recover during competition or training – they need more rest than adults.
- Advice is given on how to improve or possibly increase nutrition.
- Coaches must be highly tolerant and understanding to performers who are experiencing behavioural and physical changes.

3.6 General Recommendations

Overall improvement in physical performance comes from the body's adaptation to the loads imposed on it during intensive training. Only regular training leads to this adaptation and the resulting improvement, therefore good nutrition has to be maintained. An adequate diet is very important for the growing performer as the demands of puberty increase nutritional needs (see above).

Attention must be paid to eating habits for 365 days of the year, not just on competition days. What performers are looking for is a good balance of foods which will supply them with the fuels their bodies need for high-grade performance. The following suggestions provide a guideline to the balance of carbohydrates, fibre, fats, proteins, vitamins and minerals needed by the body. It must be remembered that when it comes to nutrition, what is good for a performer is just as good for an active coach.

High-carbohydrate Foods

The primary function of carbohydrate based foods is to supply energy for all bodily functions. It is, therefore, logical that a performer will need to increase energy intake to meet the extra demands from exercise.

Confectionery or sweet foods must not be relied on solely to provide carbohydrate in the diet. For breakfast, muesli or cereals should be opted for in preference to sweetened cereal products. In addition, fresh fruit juice, tea or coffee will maintain fluid levels. If breakfast is missed because of training, a simple carbohydrate muesli or fruit and nut bar is an ideal replacement. Bread consumption can be increased but care must be taken not to add too much fat. The consumption of plenty of fresh or frozen vegetables (particularly root varieties and green leafy vegetables), potatoes, fresh and dried fruit (particularly citrus fruits), cereals (eg pasta, rice, muesli) and pulses (eg peas, all types of beans, lentils) should be encouraged. All of these foods are high in carbohydrate, fibre, vitamins and minerals without added fat.

Fat

Performers should be encouraged to reduce the overall amount of fat (particularly saturated fats) in the diet. Fat should never be totally omitted, as some are essential to normal bodily function (eg myelin sheaths for motor nerves, page 26).

Performers should try to reduce any visible fat (eg butter, oils, lard, fat on meat) and non-visible fats (eg milk, dairy produce, eggs, mayonnaise, sausages, pâté, batter, pies and pastry). Low-fat spreads, semi-skimmed milk and low-fat cheese are healthier alternatives along with grilling, stir-frying or steaming food. Try to avoid adding unnecessary fat to a dish (eg gravy, sauces). Natural yoghurt or citrus fruit juice can be used as a substitute for mayonnaise and oil based dressings.

Protein

There is no need to eat large amounts of red meat; most recommendations suggest lean red meat once or twice a week is acceptable. Lean or white meats (eg chicken or turkey) are better than high-fat meats such as lamb, beef, pork and duck.

Table 7: Fats

Visible Fats

Butter, margarine, Outline
Lard, suet, dripping
Oils, vegetable, fish
Fatty meat, pork crackling and scratchings
Skin on chicken and duck

Non-visible Fats

Meat: beef, pork, lamb, bacon, ham, duck
Oily fish, mackerel, sardines, pilchards,
salmon, herrings
Meat pies, pasties, sausages, burgers, pâtés, salami,
pork pies
Cheese (except curd, cottage and low fat types)
Whole milk, cream, creamy puddings, cheesecakes
Nuts, olives, avacado pears
Chips, crisps, fried foods
Mayonnaise, peanut butter

Low fat alternatives:
Skimmed milk, skimmed milk products, low-fat
cheeses (eg cottage, curd, Tendale, Shape), low-fat
spreads (eg Gold, Outline), use natural yoghurt
instead of cream, white meats – poultry (remove the
skin), white fish (eg plaice, cod, coley, sole,
shellfish), crustaceans (eg crab).

Table 8: Proteins

Vegetable Proteins

Pulses, lentils, peas
Beans: haricot, mung, butter, baked beans
Nuts and seeds
Bread, potatoes, cereals, pasta, rice

Animal Proteins

Meat, poultry, offal
Fish, shellfish
Milk, cheese, yoghurt
Eggs

Vegetable proteins are high in carbohydrate
and fibre.
Animal proteins tend to be high in fat and salt.

The claims by manufacturers regarding protein supplements need to be
considered carefully. Analysing the content label of foodstuffs will often give a
good idea of the relative values:

Protein supplement sachet (18g):   Protein = 6.2g
Carbohydrate = 8.9g

Baked beans (225g can):   Protein = 11.3g
Carbohydrate = 29.5g

The baked beans not only offer more protein but also more fuel. It must be noted,
however, that excess amino acids may be converted and stored as fat. There is
evidence to suggest that amino acids can produce toxic reactions in humans.

Fluid Intake

Performers must maintain a high fluid level as part of the normal diet. It is important not to become dehydrated before or during any training session. It is advisable to consume liquid before training sessions and small amounts during the session. Research has shown cool drinks empty more rapidly from the stomach with no noticeable signs of cramp.

Thirst is not a good indication of dehydration and should be avoided by drinking regularly. Over-sugary drinks can lead to dehydration and should be avoided (eg concentrated juices and squash). Water and diluted squash are excellent ways to replace body fluids quickly. This basically constitutes an isotonic drink, as the concentration of simple sugars and electrolytes corresponds to those in the blood making it easily absorbed by the bloodstream. The advantage of such drinks is that dehydration is prevented by replacing the liquid (water) lost from sweating.

The use of strengthened carbohydrate replacement drinks needs to be closely monitored. These may be used after intense activity to refuel depleted glycogen stores when appropriate foods are not available.

A high calorie intake is needed during events where performers have prolonged energy requirements (eg cyclists in the *Tour de France* or marathon canoeists). In these circumstances, carbohydrate replacement drinks are ideal. In the past, performers have suffered by using high carbohydrate replacement drinks at the onset of an endurance event when glycogen stores are already full. Excess use of these drinks can lead to dehydration and a decrease in performance. A more appropriate method is to use isotonic drinks initially, interspersed with lower concentration (5%) carbohydrate drinks, as they are rapidly absorbed into the bloodstream and are similar in concentration to the blood itself. During ultra-endurance events such as the *Ironman Triathlon*, the consumption of higher concentration carbohydrate drinks has been used to assist in the refuelling of depleted energy stores.

Snacks

Meals should not be restricted to traditional mealtimes as this can result in eating far too much three times a day. A suggestion is to eat smaller and more frequent meals throughout the day.

Mid-morning or afternoon snacks can help, particularly when training in the early evening. This is often referred to as grazing and performers would leave no more than five hours (maximum) between meals, preferably four hours. For example, many young performers will eat at lunchtime (approximately 12:30 pm) and then go to training (early evening (approximately 17:00 pm) without refuelling – energy stores will be partially depleted before they start training.

Young performers still at school or college should be encouraged to take snacks with them to school or college to be eaten between meals.

Refuelling

The refuelling process should start as soon after training as possible as the muscle's capacity to refuel is greatest during the first hour after training. It is important that the coach and performer ensure high carbohydrate snacks and meals are readily available to promote rapid refuelling.

Rest Days

Rest days are important to give the body time to benefit from training and allow the process of adaption and recovery from the stresses of training. A sensible diet must be maintained during this time. Above all, carbohydrate stores must be refuelled adequately (page 65).

TASK

To highlight the need for good nutrition, it may be useful to think about each of the recommendations (previously mentioned) in relation to your sport and its demands.

Diet in Preparation for Competition

A new diet should not be tried in the week prior to competition. Performers should rehearse their competition diet during training sessions and minor competitions to ensure it suits their needs. Although there is little evidence to suggest that greatly elevated stores of glycogen in the body will improve performance in every sport, it appears that low glycogen stores are always a disadvantage.

Good preparation ensures the body should have at least its normal glycogen stores prior to competition.

This can be achieved by:

- tapering training (ie by gradually reducing the volume of training)
- increasing carbohydrate intake.

In the week before competition, the elite performer should maintain a carbohydrate rich diet and reduce training to increase the body's carbohydrate (glycogen) stores. Eating more carbohydrate than normal as training is tapered will result in considerably greater than normal glycogen stores. There is no evidence that these would be disadvantageous in any activity, although it may be found that there is a slight increase in body weight.

Those performers who need to make weight to stay within a specific competition class may have to monitor their carbohydrate intake more carefully. Eating large meals should be avoided and smaller, more frequent high-carbohydrate meals consumed instead. Plenty of fluids must be taken during the pre-competition week to ensure full hydration before competing. Gradual increases in carbohydrate intake throughout the week should be made, as last minute cramming does not work. Prior preparation and planning is the key to success in all respects.

Competition day

A new diet must not be tried. If the competition starts early in the morning, performers should be advised to eat a carbohydrate rich meal the evening before and appropriate breakfast arrangements must be made. It is advisable to eat a breakfast with a high G-I and plenty of fluids. Low G-I carbohydrates may be of better value in terms of maintaining a stable blood sugar level. This is due to the slower rate at which these starch based foods are digested. However, adequate time must be given to digest any food before competing, even if this means eating earlier than usual.

Coping with competition

Competition tension must be coped with sensibly. Anxiety will tend to slow the rate at which food moves out of the stomach, therefore allowances must be made. If normal food cannot be tolerated, carbohydrate drinks are a useful alternative. Pre-competition eating and drinking habits are very specific to the individual; performers will find a routine which best suits them.

Fluid and food intake during competition

Performers must maintain adequate fluid levels so that the performance is not impaired. Insufficient fluid intake during exercise will rapidly limit the capacity to lose heat through sweating and will result in overheating. It is therefore important to take fluid before and during competition, preferably by sipping small amounts regularly. Plain water or a dilute electrolyte/glucose solution will maintain fluid levels.

If the competition continues throughout the day, fluids and high G-I carbohydrates (eg piece of fruit, muesli snack bar) should be taken in small amounts in between performances. The fluid will prevent dehydration and the carbohydrate helps to maintain glycogen levels. Commercial drinks have been developed for this purpose. Refuelling is essential before, during and after training and competition to enhance recovery.

Gastro-intestinal problems

Stomach troubles (eg diarrhoea) are common complaints during competition, particularly when abroad. Dehydration can rapidly occur, losing both water and important electrolytes from the body. It is unwise to compete in this state. Peak performance will not be attained and the health of the performer may be in serious danger. In such cases, priority must be to re-establish normal fluid and energy (if permitted) levels. Plenty of fluids must

Guidelines for competing overseas:

- Drink only bottled (sealed) water when competing overseas to avoid any possible contamination (avoid ice water or ice cubes).
- Avoid common foods associated with diarrhoea (ie shellfish, undercooked or spicy foods).
- Wash and peel fruit.
- Eat familiar foods.
- Eat in places where the standard of hygiene appears acceptable – snacks from roadside vendors should be avoided.
- Avoid alcohol and unusual foods.
- When abroad it is also worthwhile to take a suitable supply of non-perishable items (eg muesli bars) which will not deteriorate in the heat.

TASK

Using the information from this chapter, identify situations in the past where inadequate diet preparation before, during and after competition affected overall performance. Think about forthcoming competitions and how you can best plan and prepare to achieve maximum performance gains.

be sipped continuously throughout the day, ideally a dilute glucose/electrolyte solution. Prevention of gastro-intestinal problems is better than cure. Although it is almost impossible to avoid the more virulent forms of digestive disorder for which some parts of the world are so justly famous, a reasonable amount of care can greatly lessen the risks.

3.7 Weight Loss

Weight can be lost by:

- changing eating habits

- increasing activity levels

- changing eating habits **and** increasing activity levels (generally the most effective method of losing weight).

The aim of all reducing diets is to restrict the food intake so the body's fat reserve (the long-term energy storage depot) is gradually reduced while the normal functions of the body are maintained. However, under severe dieting, the weight lost over the initial few weeks is likely to be the body's carbohydrate and fluid reserves, rather than fat. Without either of these, training will be both extremely difficult and tiring.

Traditional Approaches

Most traditional weight reduction programmes advocate avoiding sweet foods (eg cakes, biscuits, confectionery), potatoes and bread. Although such a diet does indeed reduce overall energy intake, it does so by drastically reducing the carbohydrate intake. Consequently, the ability to maintain muscle glycogen levels is severely impaired, along with the capacity to exercise.

Alternative Approaches

The best approach is to reduce the energy intake, while making certain that the nutrient density (in particular the carbohydrate intake) is kept high. While all the foods should be relatively low in energy, they should also be high in carbohydrate, vitamins, minerals and trace elements, rather than simply high in fibre.

A successful reducing diet should be high in carbohydrate and low in fat. This is easily achieved by removing all visible fat from the diet, substituting high-fat foods with low-fat foods and eating complex carbohydrates. If the diet is already very low in fat, then the only remedy is to reduce the overall quantity of food being consumed (and increase exercise).

A Way of Life

Ideally, a long-term weight reduction programme should not be a diet but a healthy way of life. Habits should be adjusted to provide a well-balanced diet with slightly smaller quantities. This should be maintained without reverting to previous poor eating habits that caused the original weight gain.

Realistic Weight Loss

A realistic target is to lose at most one kilogram (2.2lbs) per week. The best weight loss may be slow but it should also be permanent. By improving eating habits combined with a regular training programme, sensible weight loss may be achieved.

Alcohol

This should be consumed with care when trying to lose weight. Weight for weight, alcohol contains nearly twice as many calories as carbohydrate or protein.

Weight Balance

Once a desirable weight has been achieved, the new and improved eating habits should be maintained. Gradually slightly more should be eaten until there is no further weight loss and then the amount of food needed to maintain both body weight and training can be established. If body weight starts to increase again, return to the weight-losing routine until an acceptable balance is achieved.

Eating Related Disorders

Weight loss can become an obsession. Care must be taken not to over-emphasise the benefits of being slim and signs of anorexia nervosa or bulimia should always be investigated. Coaches must not underestimate their influence and responsibility in this area.

3.8 Making Weight

The term *making weight* means adjusting weight to come within a particular class (eg flyweight, heavyweight). If performers are competing in sports with weight categories, particular care must be taken when attempting to make weight, whether make in this context means adding or removing the grams or ounces.

Rapid weight loss should be avoided. Performers should not compete in a class that is well below their natural weight. If they always have to lose five kilograms or more to make weight, they should reconsider their weight class. A performer's weight during training should be relatively close to competition weight (within 2–3kg) with the final weight achieved gradually. Current research has shown that boxers have an increased susceptibility to brain damage from a blow to the head if they have endured significant weight loss prior to a bout due to the effects of dehydration.

Dehydration/fasting routines should be avoided because they will always result in large decreases in body fluids and glycogen, making it difficult to rehydrate and refuel sufficiently before competing. The refuelling and rehydration process after such routines will take several days, therefore performance will inevitably be impaired. As a general rule, the maximum weight a lean individual can lose without affecting fluid and glycogen stores is around one kg per week. Therefore performers should be within their class weight seven to ten days before competing, with three days being considered the absolute minimum.

If a fasting and dehydration routine has been adopted in order to make the weight, then the performer must at least try to make up some of the deficit of water, electrolytes and carbohydrate. This routine may have left the performer with undesirable side effects such as:

- severe dehydration
- liver glycogen deficiency leading to low blood glucose levels
- minimal stores of muscle glycogen
- tiredness, nausea and dizziness.

These are hardly the best conditions in which to compete. The use of diuretics (substances promoting fluid loss) should be avoided at all costs. These not only impair performance but can endanger overall health.

3.9 Gaining Weight

Weight can be gained by increasing the amount of either fat or muscle within the body. Gains in body fat are easy to achieve but gains in muscle mass are only attained as a result of adaptation to intensive training. Eating a high-protein diet will not result in increases in muscle. Any protein consumed in excess of requirements will simply be stored as fat or excreted from the body. The common practice of eating large amounts of meat, dairy produce and eggs can be expensive and is possibly detrimental to both health and performance for two reasons:

- Abnormal eating habits are established which will be difficult to alter in later life and may increase the risk of coronary heart disease.

- Eating high-protein foods leaves little appetite for those important high-carbohydrate foods. Without adequate energy intake and glycogen reserves, the performer will not be able to train to full potential and the adaptation (in this case muscle gain) will be minimal.

The best approach is to consume a high-carbohydrate diet which will ensure that glycogen stores are full before each training session. By meeting the demands of the increasing volume and quality of training, muscle mass should increase. If performers fail to refuel adequately between sessions, they will not be able to maintain their training schedules. This is often associated with constant tiredness and the smell of pear-drops on the breath or urine. This is a sure sign that the body is not receiving enough carbohydrate.

If complex carbohydrates are included in a performer's diet in the form of grain produce, pulses, legumes and nuts, the overall intake of essential amino acids naturally increases, along with carbohydrate, vitamins and minerals. While it is preferable to try to limit weight gain so that only muscle mass is increased, this is rarely achieved in practice.

It is probably easier to accept the small increases in fat stores associated with weight gain and then to reduce these once the desired muscle mass has been attained. However, the need to gain weight should not be used as an excuse to overeat.

3.10 Energy Systems

The energy made available from the digestion of food can either be:

- stored as glycogen in the liver and blood or as fat in the body
- released as heat energy through increased heat production
- converted to mechanical energy through muscular contraction allowing the body to move and function.

Adenosine Triphosphate (ATP) is an important organic molecule found in all living organisms. The energy stored in ATP is important to the body because it provides the energy used in nearly all of the chemical reactions within the cells. All muscle activity is fuelled by ATP which provides the energy for the movement of the protein filaments (Section 1.12 page 24).

$$\text{ATP} \rightarrow \text{ADP} + \text{Pi} + \text{energy}$$
$$\text{(phosphate)} \quad \text{to do work}$$

ATP is stored in the myosin heads and is the only chemical capable of producing this energy fast enough and in sufficient quantities to maintain activity. Due to its unstable nature, only the amount to fuel about one second of intense muscular activity can be stored. Therefore it has to be reformed (resynthesised) continually from **Adenosine Diphosphate (ADP)**, located in the muscles, to maintain muscular contraction. The energy for the resynthesis of ATP comes from three different systems dependent both on the intensity of exercise and the time available. The three energy systems are the:

- phosphagen system (ATP – PC)
- anaerobic glycolytic system
- aerobic energy system (oxidative).

The three energy systems rarely work independently. In every muscle contraction there is a contribution from each, depending on the overall energy requirements. It may help to look at the contribution of the three energy systems in relation to the duration of the event, which is shown in Figure 33.

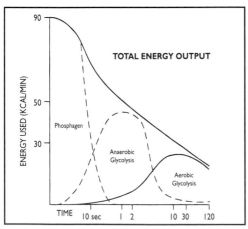

Figure 33: Graph of energy released over time

Phosphagen (ATP – PC) Energy System

The energy source is provided by the breakdown of creatine phosphate (CP) within the muscle fibres.

$$ADP + CP \rightarrow Creatine + ATP \rightarrow energy$$
$$(creatine \qquad\qquad to\ do$$
$$phosphate) \qquad\qquad work$$

The phosphagen energy system provides energy for explosive movements or short bursts of activity and lasts for about ten seconds (eg those that occur in team games). Adenosine Triphosphate (ATP) is produced from the breakdown of stored phosphocreatine. The amount of stored ATP is limited to about one second of high intensity exertion and does not appear to increase with training. Phosphocreatine stores can increase by up to 30% after training.

Unfortunately training effects are short lived so this type of training must be carried out during the competitive season. Phosphagen stores are half recovered in 30 seconds and fully recovered in five minutes, provided the performer rests. This explains why repeated short sprints with appropriate recovery are possible and why a 100 metre sprinter for example, can run a number of heats of the event on the same day, yet maintain quality performances.

Anaerobic Glycolytic Energy System

This system relies on the breakdown of glycogen stored in the muscle to provide energy for limited periods (2–3 minutes) of high intensity work.

ADP + glucose → ATP + lactate → energy to do work

TASK

Lactate accumulation can drastically limit performance and will determine the duration of high intensity activity in any sport (eg rowing). Try this simple exercise but remember to warm-up first:

- Run as fast as possible for 400m.

- Rest for 15 seconds and repeat.

After the first effort, lactate will accumulate in the active muscles; the short rest period will then help to remove some of the excess lactate acid. Due to the build up of lactate in the working muscles, the capability of these muscles will be drastically reduced and the quality of the second effort will be somewhat less than the first one.

Lactate is produced as a metabolic intermediary which leads to muscle fatigue if allowed to accumulate. Periods of lower intensity exercise provide the opportunity to convert lactate into energy for further activity.

Anaerobic glycolysis is the main anaerobic energy system. Stored carbohydrates (blood glucose or glycogen stores from the muscles and liver) are broken down to release energy and lactic acid (via pyruvic acid). Lactic acid immediately dissociates (breaks down) into lactate plus hydrogen ions. In general, the build-up of these hydrogen ions contributes to fatigue – directly by inhibiting muscular contraction and indirectly by reducing intramuscular pH. The lactate in the muscles is:

- recycled back to pyruvate within the muscle cell which then enters the aerobic cycle

- diffused out of the cell where some may be taken up by neighbouring fibres, especially slow twitch fibres which may not be engaged in vigorous activity

- diffused from the muscle into the bloodstream and delivered to the heart, kidneys and liver; heart muscle cannot generate lactate but can use it as a fuel by converting it back to pyruvate.

The efficiency of lactate clearance as performance increases is shown in Figure 34. Elite runners can achieve greater running speeds at relatively low blood lactate levels as their systems become more efficient in the clearance of blood lactate.

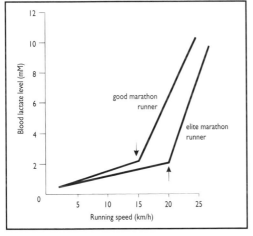

Figure 34: Efficiency of lactate removal

Aerobic Oxidative Energy System

This is the long-term energy system providing energy beyond 2–3 minutes up to several hours, at medium to low intensity.

$$\text{Glucose/fatty acids} + Pi + ADP + O_2 \rightarrow ATP$$
$$\downarrow$$
$$\text{energy to do work}$$
$$+$$
$$CO_2 / H_2O$$

Energy is converted from the breakdown of food products in the mitochondria of the muscle to produce energy. Carbon dioxide and water are produced as metabolites and absorbed into the bloodstream and removed.

TASK

Fatigue will occur quite rapidly if there is no oxygen available to resynthesise ATP. This can be shown by performing the following exercise using the press-up:

1 Perform as many press-ups as possible and record the number.

2 Repeat but time each lift at two second intervals (with arms bent).

3 Repeat but extend rest interval to 20 seconds between lifts.

Fatigue will occur fairly rapidly with a two second delay but the total number of lifts achieved will increase. If the delay is increased to 20 seconds, fatigue is noticeably delayed and the number of lifts increased. This is due to the time available for sufficient amounts of ATP to be resynthesised in the working muscle to fuel the action.

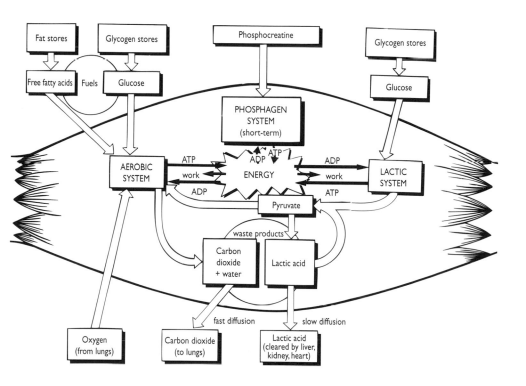

Figure 35: Flowchart of aerobic and anaerobic energy systems

3.11 Summary

Eating habits greatly affect the provision of energy to the working muscles. It is the contribution of specific nutrients that will determine the energy available for exercise. A well balanced, energy dense diet will aid any training programme and ultimately improve performance. ATP is generated through three energy systems:

- ATP – PC system
- Anaerobic glycolytic system
- Aerobic, oxidative system.

These energy systems form an energy continuum in that no one system runs independently of the others.

There are several sources of information for further study:

Bean, A (2000) **The complete guide to sports nutrition.** London, A & C Black. ISBN 0 713653 89 2

Burke, L (1996) **The complete guide to food for sports performance.** Sydney, Allen & Unwin. ISBN 1 863739 16 5

Clark, N (1997) **Sports nutrition guidebook.** Champaign IL, Human Kinetics. ISBN 0 873227 30 1

Crosland, J (1999) **Fuelling Performers.** Leeds, National Coaching Foundation. ISBN 1 902523 23 7*

Department of Health (1994) **Dietary reference values for food energy and nutrients for the United Kingdom**. London, HMSO. ISBN 0 11 321397 2

Eisenman, P, Johnson, S and Benson, J (1990) **Coaches guide to nutrition and weight control.** Champaign IL, Leisure Press. ISBN 0 88011 365 0

Hickson, J F and Wolinsky, I (1993) **Nutrition in exercise and sport.** 2nd edition, Boca Raton FLA, CRC Press. ISBN 0 8493 7911 3

Williams, C, and Devlin, I (1992) **Foods, nutrition and sports performance**. London, E & F N Spon. ISBN 0 419 17890 2

In addition, the **sports coach UK** workshop **Fuelling Performers** is recommended. Dates and venues are available from your nearest Regional Training Unit for Sport or home country office (see page 160).

---

* Complimentary with the **sports coach UK** workshop **Fuelling Performers** or available from **Coachwise 1st4sport** (0113-201 5555 or visit www.1st4sport.com).

TASK

The following tasks will help you analyse your diet and identify areas for improvement. How can you adjust your current diet to optimise performance taking into account the sport, duration and intensity of training and competition?

1 Which of the three energy systems does your sport use predominately?

2 Record and analyse your diet over one week. Is it balanced (eg are you eating a good balance of nutrients)? How can you improve it to increase energy levels (if required) and reduce fats? Note the effects this may have on performance.

3 Test your approach to nutrition by answering the following questionnaire on eating habits for coaches and performers.

   1 Compared with average males and females, would you describe yourself as:

   a underweight

   b the correct weight for your size and sport

   c overweight.

   2 Would you describe yourself as:

   a somebody who is very concerned about the foods you eat – you only use natural foods from healthfood shops, and adhere to a strict set of eating habits?

   b somebody who believes you can eat what you like and it will have little effect on your performance or health?

   c someone who honestly appreciates the possible benefits of eating sensibly and are reasonably careful in what you eat?

3   In your normal diet, how often do you eat one or more of the following types of food: beef, pork, lamb, cream, pies, pastries, milk, cheese, butter?

   a   Not at all or only sparingly.

   b   Occasionally.

   c   Most days.

4   Do you have a sweet tooth and use sugar (of any kind) in cooking and add it to your food?

   a   No – never.

   b   Yes – but only occasionally.

   c   Yes – all the time.

5   Do you think you eat a diet that is high in dietary fibre?

   a   Yes – because you eat a lot of high-fibre foods.

   b   Yes – because you put bran on your breakfast cereal.

   c   No – because you do not like high-fibre foods like wholemeal bread.

6   Do you use beans, pulses and legumes as part of your normal diet?

   a   Yes – frequently as both main meals and side dishes or snacks.

   b   Yes – but mainly as side dishes or snacks, not main meals.

   c   Not really – only used rarely as a side dish or snack.

7   Do you regularly use vitamin pills, tonics and potions to supplement your normal diet?

   a   No – you believe that you can get all the nutrients in your normal diet.

   b   Yes – you just use a single multivitamin preparation.

   c   Yes – you really believe in them and use several different types.

8   How frequently do you use convenience foods as part of your normal diet?

  ☐   a   Not at all – you think they are harmful.

  ☐   b   Occasionally – mainly frozen vegetables, meat and fish.

  ☐   c   Most of the time – you live out of the freezer on processed foods.

9   Are you conscious of the daily amount and type of carbohydrates you eat?

  ☐   a   No – eat anything put in front of you regardless of content.

  ☐   b   Not really – although you try to eat more complex carbohydrate foods.

  ☐   c   Yes – you are very particular in the type and amount of each carbohydrate and are conscious of achieving an appropriate balance.

10 Do you have a varied and balanced diet?

  ☐   a   Only occasionally, depending on what is in the cupboard.

  ☐   b   Just lunch-times; breakfast and dinner is always the same.

  ☐   c   Yes, you always plan a varied, balanced menu each week.

11 Do you have any say in the foods that you eat?

  ☐   a   Yes – you choose the majority of foods that you eat.

  ☐   b   Yes – within the confines of your budget and family constraints.

  ☐   c   Not at all – you simply eat what is put in front of you.

12 How often do you adapt recipes to make them more healthy (eg replace cream with fromage frais or yoghurt, reduce visible fat content)?

    a   Always adapt recipes to reduce fat content and increase complex carbohydrate content.

    b   A little bit – enough to ensure fat content is not excessive but you are not obsessive.

    c   Never – you always follow them regardless of content.

How did you score?

1: a = 1, b = 2, c = 0	5: a = 2, b = 1, c = 0	9: a = 2, b = 1, c = 0
2: a = 1, b = 0, c = 2	6: a = 2, b = 1, c = 0	10: a = 2, b = 1, c = 0
3: a = 1, b = 2, c = 0	7: a = 2, b = 1, c = 0	11: a = 2, b = 1, c = 0
4: a = 1, b = 2, c = 0	8: a = 1, b = 2, c = 0	12: a = 2, b = 1, c = 0

Scoring:

0–8
Your eating habits could certainly be improved. Adopting some of the suggestions given in this chapter may have quite an impact on your performance, as well as on your health.

8–15
Some of your better eating habits are balanced by others which tend to reduce the overall standard of your diet. A few alterations and a bit of effort would make considerable improvements in the quality of your diet. Could certainly try harder.

15–24
Your eating habits are generally good but not perfect. Even a score of 24+ may only reflect the fact that you are into nutrition at the moment. Unless you stick with these eating habits, you may find that your performance will start to deteriorate.

Comment on answers

The value of this questionnaire is not simply in giving good or bad advice to increase diet awareness among performers. The answers in most instances are pretty obvious, in fact some of the questions are loaded to make a point. Question 1 raises the subject of being overweight. Question 2 is intended to introduce a commonsense approach to nutrition – not being either fanatical or apathetic about it. Questions 3–6 raise the point about energy sources and the different types of fat and carbohydrate in the diet – how to make sure your carbohydrate is reasonably high. Question 7 introduces the value or otherwise of vitamin supplementation. The potential value of frozen foods versus processed convenience foods is raised in Question 8. Finally, Questions 9–12 illustrate the problems associated with trying to improve eating habits. Fussy eaters will find it difficult to accept new foods into their diet. Eating away from home for most of the time will tend to restrict the possible improvements you can make. If you do not take any interest in the foods you eat, how can you expect to improve your eating habits? Question 12 should not be overlooked. Everybody should be able to cook well enough to eat what they want and not be forced to survive on fast foods.

SECTION TWO
Fitness Components and Training

Introduction

Section Two deals with the components of fitness and the effects of training in maximising performance potential.

- **Chapter Four** includes information and guidance on the specific endurance needs of performers and the adaptations which occur as a result of endurance training.

- **Chapter Five** investigates the role of strength, speed and power within all sports, the effects of training on specific muscles and the relevance of muscle fibre type and distribution.

- **Chapter Six** identifies the important role of flexibility training in the achievement of sporting potential and avoidance of injury.

Although each fitness component is considered in separate chapters, it is important to recognise the importance of a balanced training programme which reflects the relative contributions of each component and the specific demands of the sport.

Each chapter offers information panels to help relate material to your sport together with final tasks to enhance your understanding. This section will help coaches and performers to develop their knowledge of the components of fitness in relation to specific sports and assist in the designing of effective and efficient training programmes to maximise performance and limit injury.

CHAPTER FOUR:
Endurance

4.0 Introduction

Endurance is a term that describes two separate but related concepts:

- Muscular endurance
- Cardiorespiratory endurance.

Whereas muscular endurance refers to the ability of individual muscles, cardiorespiratory endurance relates to the body as a whole. Specifically, it relates to the body's ability to sustain prolonged, rhythmical exercise. This type of endurance is typified by the cyclist, distance runner or endurance swimmer who can complete long distances at a fairly fast pace. A person's cardiorespiratory endurance is closely related to the development of his/her cardiovascular and respiratory systems, and therefore, aerobic development.

Each sport has differing energy demands classified broadly as **aerobic** (with oxygen, long-term) and **anaerobic** (without oxygen, short-term). Four hundred metre runners, for example, require a high anaerobic capacity, while marathon runners depend heavily on aerobic metabolism. Football and tennis players will use both systems combining repeated explosive bursts of energy interspersed with periods of lower intensity exercise. To show how

endurance can be developed in sport and how the body adapts to endurance based training, it is important to have an understanding of the energy systems (which were discussed in Section 3.10 page 86).

4.1 Aerobic Endurance

The aerobic energy system is completely dependent on the supply of oxygen by the oxygen transport system. Oxygen arriving in muscle blood capillaries diffuses to the myoglobin (muscle storage protein for oxygen) and mitochondria where aerobic glycolysis occurs. In aerobic glycolysis, glycogen is broken down to pyruvic acid in an eight-step process (and this still occurs when oxygen is not present). The presence of oxygen ensures that pyruvic acid is not converted to lactic acid but is converted to carbon dioxide and water, having passed through the Krebs Cycle and oxidative phosphorylation (also known as the *electron transport chain*).

Aerobic energy is not only important to aerobic endurance performers – many other activities have a large aerobic element (eg multiple sprint sports such as rugby, squash, hockey). Even in activities which are essentially anaerobic (eg 400 metre running, hurdling), aerobic training is crucial because a well developed aerobic system delays the onset of lactate accumulation and fatigue.

A performer's aerobic power or work capacity is known as the $\dot{V}O_2$ max (the maximum volume of oxygen which can be used per minute) and is measured in millilitres per minute. Since body weight varies between performers, it is usually given per kg of body weight (ie ml/min/kg). In some sports absolute $\dot{V}O_2$ is expressed rather than $\dot{V}O_2$ per kg body weight (eg rowing, cycling). Elite performers from the same sport would not be expected to score the same on a $\dot{V}O_2$ max test, as there are a number of individual differences which affect the rate of oxygen uptake:

- **Genetic composition** of the muscle fibres will be the major cause of individual differences. It is believed approximately 93% of an individual's $\dot{V}O_2$ max is determined by genetics, although controversy exists about whether this figure may be too high. Individuals predisposed to low aerobic capacities will be unable to improve their $\dot{V}O_2$ max dramatically through training. It is widely accepted that endurance performers (and in fact sprinters) are born and not made.

- The **sex** of the performer is also significant, as males generally have a higher maximum due to the differences in body fat measurements and the higher haemoglobin status compared with females. Males have a greater percentage of muscle mass and larger hearts than females.

- **Age** affects an individual's $\dot{V}O_2$ max. It will reduce with age along with the maximal heart rate.

- **Time of day** affects an individual's oxygen consumption. Research has indicated that some individuals obtain higher values in the evening compared with the morning (values may differ by as much as 3–5%).

Although an individual's $\dot{V}O_2$ max appears to be predetermined by genetics, age and sex, performers can train at intensities where lactate (in the blood) will accumulate to very high levels. This will train the body to become more efficient in the removal or utilisation of lactate (to energy). Therefore, training can help performers to improve their % $\dot{V}O_2$ max at which they can perform, before lactate accumulation and attendant hydrogen ions cause a reduction in performance (Figure 33, Section 3.10 page 86).

TASK

How might the aerobic capacity of endurance sports (eg marathon runners, cyclists, rowers) differ from that of other sports (eg wrestling, weight training, boxing)? Would you expect all performers to have the same values within a sport? Think about the differences in energy demand within a team (eg goalkeeper and a forward position). Who needs a greater aerobic capacity?

4.2 Muscle Fibre Type

Another factor which influences the efficiency of the body to tolerate prolonged aerobic activity is the muscle fibre type. Chapter One referred to the three types of fibre (page 28) but it is the ratio of slow to fast twitch fibres in each individual that is important to endurance training.

Individuals with a higher percentage of fast twitch fibres are more likely to excel at power events as fast fibres contract faster and without the presence of oxygen. In contrast, higher concentrations of slow twitch fibres favour endurance events as they more readily utilise the oxygen supply from the blood and are slow to fatigue. The ratio of muscle fibre types is genetically determined but current research has shown that endurance training can cause a shift in the characteristics of some of the fibres.

4.3 Muscle Responses to Endurance Training

In order to benefit from an increase in oxygen supply, the muscles must be capable of utilising the oxygen to release energy. Physiological adaptations occur in the muscle as a result of endurance training which promotes increased efficiency in energy provision:

- **Muscle blood flow**. The number and density of the muscle cell capillaries increases with aerobic training providing a greater surface area for oxygen exchange. Aerobically trained muscle will have up to 50% more capillaries than untrained muscle.

- Increases in **myoglobin** occur as muscle tissue increases with training. Myoglobin attracts oxygen away from the haemoglobin in the blood, through the capillary walls and into the muscles (ie it increases the rate of oxygen movement into the muscle fibres). The levels of myoglobin play an important role in the short-term storage of oxygen.

- **Mitochondria** refers to the specialised structures which are the sites for the chemical release of energy and can be regarded as the power houses of the muscle cell. Experiments have shown that following aerobic training there is an increase in both the size and number of mitochondria. The greatest increases occur in cells of aerobic fast twitch fibres followed by the aerobic slow twitch fibres. Even the anaerobic fast twitch muscle cells show a considerable increase in mitochondria. This increase complements the increase in capillaries and oxygen rich myoglobin which allows more fuel to reach the muscles and be fully utilised.

- The concentration of certain **enzymes** for energy conversion in the muscle cell also increases enhancing chemical reactions.

4.4 Training for Aerobic Endurance

The heart, lungs, blood vessels and blood are the basic elements of the oxygen transport system (Section 2.1 page 38). The heart shows the greatest response to training and can be easily monitored by checking the performer's heart rate (eg pulse).

Aerobic training is part of almost every sport but it is important to understand the reasons why it is included, to ensure it is carried out effectively.

Training for aerobic endurance is important for three main reasons:

- It is a fundamental part of any sport and training programme, and acts as a foundation on which to build other fitness parameters

- It will improve the efficiency and effectiveness of the oxygen transport system

- It reduces recovery time.

The aim of aerobic endurance training is to raise the heart rate to an appropriate level and sustain it for an appropriate period of time. The problem lies in detecting the appropriate levels and duration.

These vary depending on the sport, age and the fitness level of the performer. As the performer improves, the frequency, duration and intensity of training should be increased to ensure progression.

4.5 Aerobic Endurance Programmes

When designing an aerobic endurance programme, it is important to consider the following training principles:

- Progressive overload
- Specificity
- Recovery
- Reversibility
- Monitoring and adaptability.

Progressive Overload

In order to increase the endurance capacity of an individual, the exercise intensity must place the body under stress. In response to this training overload, the body adapts to meet the additional demands by producing more muscle tissue or increasing the efficiency of the cardio-respiratory system. In time, the original stimulus will become a comfortable workload due to these training adaptations. Progressive overload can be achieved by controlling (usually by gradually increasing) the frequency, intensity and time (duration) of training;

- **Frequency of training** depends on the intensity and duration of each training session and the fitness level of the performer. It has been suggested that significant levels of aerobic fitness can be achieved by training four times a week. However, the optimum number will depend on each individual and the relative importance of aerobic fitness in each sport.

- **Intensity of training** – the most important aspect of aerobic training – depends on the performer's current fitness level and frequency and duration of training. It is now generally accepted that there is an **aerobic threshold** below which there is insufficient stimulus to the cardiovascular system to bring about any long-term changes.

  This threshold occurs at different heart rates for different performers and varies with age and fitness.

  Equally there is an upper limit above which the body can no longer sustain aerobic exercise and the energy contribution from anaerobic sources is such that there is a marked rise in lactate levels. This is called the **lactate threshold** and is generally between 60 and 90% of maximum heart rate.

- **Time or duration** of an aerobic training session depends on the training intensity and fitness level of the performer.[1]

---

1 This can be remembered as the FIT principle.

Training at (or just below) the lactate threshold for 20 minutes has proved very effective. It is unlikely that this intensity can be sustained for longer due to the onset of fatigue. An alternative effective training method would be to exercise at a slightly lower intensity (but still high intensity) for a longer duration. Therefore, it is important to adapt the session to meet the needs of the specific sport.

Specificity

Training must be specific, for this ensures adaptations to match the physiological demands of the sport. Aerobic training should be specific, not only to the cardiovascular system but also to the aerobic aspects of the muscles. For example, a swimmer who cycles for a large proportion of training will experience benefits to the central cardio-respiratory system (eg the heart muscle will become conditioned) but not to the specific musculature used in swimming.

Recovery

Adaptation to the increased stresses of training will only result in performance gains if sufficient and appropriate recovery periods are incorporated into training programmes. If high intensity training occurred every day without adequate recovery, there would be little or no adaptation (ie including the growth and repair of tissue).

Recovery for young performers

Growing is an exhausting business. The cumulative effect of training, lifestyle and growing can quickly drain a child's energy resources. Coaches must consider carefully the training ratios and loads, and plan adequate recovery periods – daily, weekly and monthly. It is also important to plan rest and adaptive phases into the yearly plan.

Recovery periods can also prevent overuse injuries and staleness by allowing various structures and systems of the body as well as the mind (psychological) to recuperate.

Recovery is extremely important but it does not necessarily mean rest. It is better to think of two types of recovery:

- **Active recovery** can be defined as low intensity, short duration training which promotes repair and rebuilding. It can also represent recovery time between intervals during a training session or simply days of low intensity, cross training[1].

- **Rest (inactive) recovery** represents a day off from training altogether and is especially important if the training intensity is high, and prior to competition, to ensure the energy stores are full.

Coaches and performers should become skilled in the recognition of fatigue or depletion. Good planning and organisation of recovery sessions is important to help promote adaptation and performance gains. For example, in endurance events, the primary concern would be the replenishment of fuel and fluid stores (eg rehydration and carbohydrate consumption). In contrast, in speed training (Chapter 5 page 116), recovery would probably concentrate on neurological functions (eg promoting muscle relaxation, active recovery and massage techniques). Recovery should be sport and individual specific (eg a marathon runner will not have the same recovery period as a badminton player). Sports are diverse and recovery periods must be matched to the training demands to accelerate adaptation and fully maximise performance benefits.

TASK

To help assess individual recovery rates it is useful to keep a training diary. For example, if a triathlete does high intensity sessions on consecutive days without any recovery, the energy systems will become depleted (the process of overtraining could begin). An effective training programme will maintain an overall balance and will alternate high and low intensity sessions. Recently, elite performers have found that a reduction in total training has, in fact, increased performance gains which further supports the vital role of specific rest periods in any training regime.

If possible, analyse the last four week training period in terms of recovery and training intensity. Look at performance gains and relate this to the frequency and duration of any rest periods.

[1] A term often used to describe a form of training incorporating a variety of activities (eg a runner may do some light swimming, cycling or aerobics).

Reversibility

Training responses will be lost through failure to maintain the training load. The rate of de-training is three times as slow as the training process. This is particularly significant during periods of injury where some kind of low intensity exercise should be maintained to offset the effects of de-training and maintain motivation and confidence.

Monitoring and Adaptability

All training programmes require close monitoring to maintain effectiveness and suitability. Initial plans can be adapted later to meet the specific needs of a performer and the principles of progression.

4.6 Types of Aerobic Training

Aerobic endurance training is designed to improve the efficiency and effectiveness of the cardio-respiratory system. This enables performers to sustain low to moderate intensity activities for longer durations (from 20 mins to in excess of three hours). Aerobic endurance can be improved by several types of training:

- Continuous activity
- Fartlek training
- Interval training
- Circuit training.

Continuous Activity

This involves moderate/medium intensity activity over a long duration (eg 30–45 minutes steady running at 65% of maximum heart rate, depending on current fitness level). It is used to provide the aerobic endurance base which underpins more specific and higher level fitness training.

Fartlek Training

This involves progressive variation of training intensity and duration utilising changes in speed (an example is shown in the next information panel). The variations can be designed to mirror or match performance demands. Fartlek training is useful in progressing from steady pace endurance training towards an introduction of related speed work.

> For example, the 1994 England World Cup Cricket Squad utilised Fartlek training as follows:
>
> Four mins jog – three mins steady run – two mins jog – three mins steady to include 1 x 50m fast burst every 30 secs – two mins jog – three mins steady to include 1 x 20m sprint every 30 secs – two mins jog – two mins fast – four mins jog.
>
> The bursts of speed match the distances, intensities and duration associated with demands made during a cricket game (eg bowler run-up, running between wickets).

Repetition Training

Repetition training involves repeated high-intensity training interspersed with relevant recovery intervals. It is probably the most common form of endurance training across a wide range of sports. The balance between work intensity and duration and the complementary recovery periods, determine the effectiveness of interval training. The effective use of interval training depends on the:

- duration or distance of work interval
- pace of work
- number of repetitions
- duration and activity of the rest interval.

For example, swimmers or cyclists may use repetition training when working at relatively high intensities (85–95% of maximal heart rate) for periods up to 2–3 minutes, which maximises the stress on the aerobic system with a high anaerobic element. For example, a swimmer could do a set of 6 x 200m swims at 85–90% of maximum effort, with a 20–30 second recovery interval between each swim. The set of 200m swims could then be followed by 10–15 minutes of active recovery; this type of set could be repeated another three times. This is often referred to as *lactate threshold* repetition training.

Circuit Training

Circuit training can involve low intensity and high repetition circuits or high intensity and low repetition circuits (a combination of both types of circuit can also be used). It can be used to develop aerobic endurance as well as local muscular endurance and strength. In order to promote gains in aerobic endurance, exercise circuits should be designed to place a suitable stress on the cardio-respiratory system. This involves the use of low resistance, high repetition exercises over a continuous period (20+ mins). Variables in circuit training are the same as those for repetition training.

Hockey players might incorporate appropriate exercises in circuit sessions (eg squat thrusts, sit ups, back raises, shuttle runs, dips, bicep curls, burpees, astride jumps, press ups, step ups and chin raises) which would be beneficial to different aspects of a game. Seven to ten exercises should be selected using alternate muscle groups. After 4–6 weeks the programme can be made more difficult by:

- increasing the number of reps/sets (ten per exercise initially)
- increasing time spent exercising (minimum 15–20 minutes)
- reducing recovery time.

4.7 Testing Aerobic Performance

Although the maximum oxygen uptake ($\dot{V}O_2$ max) can only be measured accurately using elaborate laboratory equipment, there are some relatively simple field tests for coaches and teachers to use which will give good estimates of $\dot{V}O_2$ max from sub-maximal tests. However, these field tests must:

- involve types of exercise which:
  - derive energy from aerobic sources
  - involve large muscle groups
- be easy to reproduce.

There are three basic types of field tests used to predict maximum oxygen uptake:

- Running tests (eg track, shuttles)
- Ergometer tests (eg cycle, ski, swim, run, treadmill)
- Stepping tests.

To gain a full picture of the performer's aerobic fitness, it may be desirable to undertake a maximal (ie to exhaustion) rather than a sub-maximal test. One of the most effective maximal predictive tests is the Multistage Fitness Test. Participants perform a series of 20 metre shuttle runs at increasingly faster speeds in time with a series of pre-recorded bleeps. They continue to run until they can no longer keep up with the pace of the bleeps. The test is designed to be progressive and maximal as the performers stop when they are running at their maximal speed but still failing to maintain the desired pace.

The shuttles are structured in progressive levels and the final shuttle achieved is identified in terms of the number of shuttles completed at a particular level. Using this value, the predicted maximum oxygen uptake can be calculated by inserting the value into a table.

The test only requires the pre-recorded audio tape, tape recorder and a measured length of 20 metres (plus turning space). It can be administered on a number of performers at once, provided each person has a partner to count the number of shuttles achieved. The test is ideal for measuring aerobic endurance for groups or performers. For further information on a range of field based tests and the interpretation of tests, you are recommended to read the **sports coach UK** home study pack *A Guide to Field Based Fitness Testing*.

TASK

The results from any test can only be used as guidelines and should be appropriate to the sport (eg a rower could be tested for aerobic endurance capacity on a cycle ergometer). The differences in energy needs between team players should be taken into consideration when planning training sessions. For example in netball, the centre court players require a greater level of aerobic endurance than the goalkeeper who is limited to one third of the court.

Consider the tests that may be appropriate to your sport and identify potential differences in results and subsequent training needs.

4.8 Lactate Threshold

The lactate threshold is defined as the point at which blood lactate begins to accumulate above resting levels during exercise of increasing intensity. During light to moderate activity, blood lactate remains only slightly above the resting level. With more intense effort, lactate accumulates more rapidly. By definition, the lactate threshold has been thought to reflect the interaction of the aerobic and anaerobic energy systems. Some researchers have suggested that the lactate threshold represents a significant shift toward anaerobic glycolysis, which forms lactate. Consequently, the sudden increase in blood lactate with increasing effort has also been referred to as the anaerobic threshold.

However, controversy surrounds the relationship of the lactate threshold to anaerobic metabolism in muscle. Muscles are likely to be producing lactate well before the lactate threshold is reached but it is being removed by other tissues. In addition, a clear breakpoint is not always apparent.

The rate of demand for ATP dictates lactate production. If that rate exceeds the performer's current ability to generate ATP, predominantly from aerobic glycolysis, Krebs Cycle and oxidative phosphorylation (ie aerobic metabolism), then more and more energy is derived from anaerobic glycolysis.

The lactate threshold is usually expressed in terms of the $\%\dot{V}O_2$ max at which it occurs. The ability to exercise at a high intensity without accumulating lactate is beneficial to the performer because lactate formation contributes to fatigue. Consequently, a lactate threshold at 80% $\dot{V}O_2$ max suggests a greater exercise tolerance than a threshold at 60% $\dot{V}O_2$ max. Generally, in two individuals with the same maximal oxygen uptake, the person with the higher lactate threshold exhibits the better endurance performance. This threshold is different for every performer depending on age and fitness. Several tests can be used to measure lactate threshold, including heart rate training zones and blood lactate sampling (facilities for blood lactate sampling are not generally available).

During continuous exercise, lactate is released from muscle fibres, diffuses, or is carried into other fibres where it is broken down and returned to working fibres for use as energy – this is termed the **lactate shuttle.** The amount of fuel supplied by lactate is equal to or greater than that supplied by glucose. Indeed, during exercise of an intensity of more than 50% VO_2 max, over 50% of the energy used by the heart is derived from lactate. It appears that many African middle and long-distance athletes are beginning to capitalise on the benefits of lactate shuttling during their competitive race as well as during their training programme. This has been illustrated in major international events where African athletes have dominated races from start to finish through varying and controlling the pace of a race.

4.9 Anaerobic Endurance

Anaerobic simply means without the presence of oxygen. In anaerobic training, the body is working so hard that all the oxygen needed cannot be supplied quickly enough to meet demand.

As intensity of effort increases above resting levels, there will come a point where not all the energy required to resynthesise ATP can be provided by the aerobic energy system. At this point a greater percentage of energy is obtained from the anaerobic system. Anaerobic endurance is, of necessity, short-term and is a supplement to the aerobic mechanism during conditions when the aerobic system cannot cope alone. The energy systems overlap into one another.

TASK

The ability to adapt training to achieve specific benefits is of particular importance. For instance, a middle distance runner may perform specific endurance sessions (long runs) on one day and a speed session (repetition sprints) the next. In this way the activity is broken down and provides effective benefits corresponding to the demands of the runner in a competition (eg the aerobic capacity would be improved and the runner's ability to take the race out fast or finish fast would be improved).

How might this method enhance performances in your sport?

However, the anaerobic system is evident in three main ways:

- At the beginning of a long run, row or similar exercise, before the aerobic system has been fully activated, a small oxygen deficit builds up. This only happens during the first 30 seconds and the deficit is rapidly repaid. While the system is catching up, the exercise seems harder and the performer often wonders if the activity can be sustained. However, once the original deficit is repaid, a steady state is reached. This second wind makes the exercise seem bearable once again. It is only during the initial part of the exercise that the muscles are operating anaerobically.

- In very explosive exercises, the action may be so short and sharp that it is over in a second or two before the oxygen transport system has the chance to be activated (eg throws and jumps in athletics, gymnastic vaults and weightlifting).

- Intense bursts of activity lasting from ten seconds to one minute are very anaerobic (eg sprints up to 600 metres, shorter swims, canoe/kayak sprint events and gymnastics).

The cost of aerobic and anaerobic training to the young performer:

- Children are less effective in their use of energy and generate less aerobic power than adults, therefore it is harder for children to perform steady exercise than it is for adults. However, children do actually tolerate steady activities better than more explosive ones.

- Children have less potential for performing explosive activities because they have smaller stores of anaerobic energy fuel and a lesser ability to use it.

- Children are not as well equipped to tolerate short bursts of strenuous activity as adults and not as well suited to short-repetition, high-intensity training often used by older performers.

Coaches must allow children to undertake a wide range of activities and only begin to specialise when they reach puberty.

4.10 Rest Intervals

The rest intervals in anaerobic interval training are very important to allow time for accumulated lactate to diffuse out of the muscles into the blood and then be removed or used as fuel. The first stage of clearing it from the muscles is the most important, especially if smaller muscle groups are being used (eg gymnasts on the pommel-horse).

When a muscle stops working, the blood flow drops off very quickly (within about 20 seconds) which locks the lactate within the muscle. However, continuation of the activity at a lower intensity will maintain good blood flow to the working muscles allowing the lactate to be removed from the muscle at a faster rate.

This is one reason why it is important always to cool-down after a hard workout. Applied to interval training the message is clear – rests should be active. Lactate levels are lower following such active rests than if the rest is completely inactive. This active rest appears to clear the muscle of lactate more quickly and cause accelerated uptake of lactate from the blood by other organs. This has implications for competition (eg squash players should stay active between games, rowers and canoeists should think in terms of clearing lactate after heats, and substitute players should not immediately sit down but take a 30-second cool-down).

4.11 Training Muscle Fibre Types

Most skeletal muscles contain both fast twitch (FT) and slow twitch (ST) fibres. The different types of fibre derive their names from the difference in their speed of action. This difference is due to the different forms of myosin which split the ATP to release energy for contraction or relaxation – FT have a fast form of myosin and ST have a slow form. This speed and type of myosin are dictated by the speed of the motor nerve for that motor unit.

In general ST fibres have high levels of aerobic (in the presence of oxygen) endurance and are very efficient at producing ATP from the oxidation of carbohydrate and fat. Therefore ST fibres are recruited during low/moderate-intensity endurance events, such as marathon running or channel swimming. FT fibres, on the other hand, have relatively poor aerobic endurance. They are better suited to perform anaerobically (without oxygen) than the ST fibres. This means their ATP is formed through anaerobic pathways, not oxidation (Section 3.10 page 87).

FT fibres are divided into FTa motor units and FTb motor units. FTa motor units generate considerably more force than ST motor units but they fatigue easily because of their limited endurance and appear to be used mainly during short, high-intensity endurance events such as running the 1500m or the 400m swim. The FTb fibres are not fully understood. They are not easily switched on by the nervous system and are used infrequently in normal, low-intensity activity but are predominantly used in highly explosive events such as 100m sprint or 50m swim.

4.12 Testing Anaerobic Performance

The **phosphagen energy system** is difficult to test. Phosphocreatine and ATP levels can be measured by muscle tissue samples or the newer technique of Nuclear Magnetic Resonance Spectroscopy (NMRS) but the equipment is enormously expensive. The usual method of gaining some knowledge of the size of this energy component in performers is to work them hard at an appropriate exercise mode and then to measure the recovery oxygen (or oxygen debt). The recovery oxygen has a fast phase (usually about two minutes) and a much longer slow phase (20–30 minutes). The fast phase is considered to be serviced by the oxygen which is used for the immediate resynthesis of

phosphocreatine. Thus, the greater the amount of oxygen absorbed by the performer during the first two minutes of activity, the greater the efficiency of the anaerobic energy system.

For the explosive sports (eg karate and gymnastics), lactate measurements and anaerobic output is tested on one of the various forms of the Wingate power test. The performer turns a very heavily loaded wheel for a total of 30 seconds with the arms or legs and the power output is recorded every five seconds in units of watts of power per kilogram of body weight.

Lactate testing can be achieved relatively easily by progressively working the performer harder and harder on the appropriate equipment (eg cycle/rowing ergometers, running machines, weight training equipment). Periodic fingertip or ear lobe blood samples are taken to measure lactate content in relation to workload. This progressive test is normally used to establish a performer's lactate threshold. It is more important to know how efficiently the lactate is being processed than simply how much is being produced. Trained performers have been shown to be able to turn it over five or even ten times faster than an untrained performer.

Lactate level checks have demonstrated that although squash players may produce high levels of lactate in a game, they seem able to remove it during play. Various shadow training routines have been shown to be at least as anaerobic as the games themselves and sometimes more so. Some games (eg volleyball, badminton) which, at recreational levels, are aerobic activities, become highly anaerobic sports at the top standard of play.

TASK

Each sport tends to have its own particular tests which incorporate a variety of movements (eg pull ups for sports requiring high upper body capability) and which measure performance capability by the number of repetitions completed in 30 or 60 seconds. If they are sport specific, valid and reliable, they should give a good indication of performance improvement.

Think about the tests you may use to indicate improvement and decide how appropriate they are in judging progression and how they assist in subsequent training programmes.

4.13 Muscular Endurance

Endurance can be described as both muscular and cardio-respiratory endurance. For sprinters endurance is the quality that allows them to sustain a high speed over the full distance of, for example, the 100m or 200m race. This is muscular endurance – the ability of a single muscle or muscle group to sustain high-intensity, repetitive or static exercise. However, a marathon runner's muscular endurance can be described as the muscle's ability to sustain prolonged, rhythmical fast-pace exercise. The exercising muscles involved in this type of muscular endurance become highly efficient in utilising and transporting oxygen. Muscular endurance depends on:

- strength
- the efficiency of the blood supply
- the muscle's ability to remove the metabolites of exercise (eg lactate).

Inevitably requirements for muscular endurance vary between sports. If the muscle is trained to perform a particular movement which directly reflects the muscle action of the sport in competition, it will be less likely to fatigue during competition. This relies on the principle of progressive overload and the adaptations that occur as a direct result.

4.14 Testing Muscular Endurance

Various tests can be used to plot an individual performer's progress and are valid as long as the technique and method are safe, done correctly and repeated. Typical procedures would include performing as many exercises as possible without interruption and noting the score for future comparison.

4.15 Fatigue

Muscle fatigue is the result of many factors, each related to the specific demands of the exercise that produce it. A significant reduction in muscle glycogen is related to fatigue during prolonged submaximal exercise (eg a cyclist working at 70% of maximum heart rate on a two hour training ride).

This is often referred to as *nutrient fatigue* and occurs even though sufficient oxygen is available to generate energy through aerobic pathways. Endurance athletes commonly refer to this fatigue as *hitting the wall*. However, during short-term maximal exercise, muscle fatigue is associated with oxygen lack and an increased level of blood and lactate in the exercising muscle. This anaerobic condition may cause drastic changes within and outside the many cells of the active muscles. These include changes to the:

- elastic component of muscle

- neuro-muscular fatigue

- relaxation fatigue

- joint fatigue.

Following an extended lay off from exercise, most people experience soreness in the exercised muscles and joints. A temporary soreness may persist for several hours immediately after unaccustomed exercise. Longer term soreness may appear later and last for three to four days (delayed onset muscle soreness). This can be due to:

- minute tears in the muscle tissue itself

- fluid retention in the tissues surrounding the muscle

- muscle spasms

- overstretching and perhaps tearing of portions of the muscle's connective tissue.

Coaches and performers should therefore use gradual progressions when beginning exercise programmes.

4.16 Summary

An appreciation of the involvement of muscle cells and the enormous complexity of the body explains why training cannot be made completely scientific for improved performance. These physical considerations alone ensure there will always be differences in the way the body responds to training or the onset of fatigue. It is important that the coach and performer understand and respect the physiological limits before embarking on specific training programmes. A knowledge of the three energy systems responsible for the provision of energy and their significance in relation to energy demand is vital in the pursuit of optimum performance. Further suggested readings include:

Bompa, TO (1999) **Periodization: theory and methodology of training.** Champaign IL, Human Kinetics. ISBN 0 880118 40 7

*Davies, J (1996) **Fitness for games players.** Leeds, National Coaching Foundation ISBN 0 947850 10 4

Leonard, J (1992) **Science of coaching swimming.** Champaign IL, Human Kinetics. ISBN 0 88011 450 9

McArdle, W, Katch, F and Katch V(2001) **Exercise physiology.** Malvern PA, Lea & Febiger. ISBN 0 781725 44 5

Newsholme, E, Leech, T and Duerter, G (1994) **Keep on running: the science of training performance.** Chichester, John Wiley. ISBN 0 471943 14 2

Noakes, T (2002) **Lore of running.** Champaign IL, Leisure Press. ISBN 0 8 73229 59 2

Reilly, T, Secher, N and Snell, P (1990) **Physiology of sports.** London, E & F N Spon. ISBN 0 419 13590 1

* Wilkinson, D and Moore, P (1995) **A guide to field based fitness testing.** Leeds, National Coaching Foundation. (Home study pack). ISBN 0 947850 55 4

Wilmore, J and Costill, D (1999) **Physiology of exercise and sport.** Champaign IL, Human Kinetics. ISBN 0 736000 84 4

* Complimentary with the **sports coach UK** workshop *Field Based Fitness Testing* or available from **Coachwise 1st4sport** (tel 0113-201 5555 or visit www.1st4sport.com).

TASK

The following tasks will help to identify the physiological demands of your sport and the endurance needs of the performers. This knowledge will enable you to develop a safe and effective training programme which fully utilises the energy sources available.

1 Identify the two different forms of endurance and how your sport utilises them. What factors would limit endurance performance? Using the knowledge gained from this chapter and personal experience, explain how certain training methods could overcome such limitations.

2 Which of the three energy systems does your sport use predominately? Analyse a training session to define which energy systems would be utilised at particular periods and explain why this happens. How would you expect your body to adapt during specific endurance training?

CHAPTER FIVE:
Strength, Speed and Power

5.0 Introduction

Each sport has a unique blend of techniques and physical requirements which in turn depend on the various components of fitness. This chapter will examine three related aspects of physical fitness and how the development of each will enhance a training programme:

- **Strength** is the ability of a muscle or muscle group to exert a force.

- **Speed** is the total distance travelled per unit of time
  (unit: metres per second).

- **Power** is the rate of performing work; the product of force and velocity
  (unit: watt).

While relatively few sporting activities depend on pure strength alone, the performer will inevitably find that an increase in strength in certain areas will be needed if performance is to improve. Additionally, an increase in speed will be of no benefit unless accompanied by increases in power. For example, at the start of a 250m sprint heat in canoeing, power is needed to pull away but any initial gains will soon be lost if the speed, power and strength of the paddle stroke are not developed.

5.1 Strength

Strength gains are achieved by training a muscle or group of muscles to exert a force against a large relative resistance. This force causes an increase in muscle tension. When repeated frequently, the muscle responds positively in a way that enables it to deliver more force. Strength is also an important quality in other fitness components such as:

- **muscular endurance** which is the capacity of the performer to carry out activity over a period of time (eg sustaining the stroke rate in rowing, strong returns in a tennis rally)

- **agility** where strength is needed to control body weight (eg complex movement sequences in gymnastics, rapid movements of an ice skater)

- **speed** where force is required to create rapid movements (eg sprinting, rapid movement to return shots in squash).

5.2 Speed

Speed is a major component in many sports, although its nature and function will often vary.

Speed depends on the relative contribution of the energy systems (Figure 33 page 86) and various forms of speed training will focus specifically on training a particular part of the energy system. Within running events, however, speed is significant in two ways and can be classified as follows:

- **Reaction speed** refers to the ability of a performer to react to a stimulus (eg reacting to the serve when receiving in tennis, to the sound of the starter's gun in sprinting). Any decrease in total response time will have a major effect on performance (response time = movement time + reaction time; NB reaction time is genetic and cannot be improved by training; movement time can be trained).

- **Running speed** is determined by the length and frequency of running stride. The muscle groups involved need to be strengthened so they can contract more powerfully and thus increase speed.

A senior 800m runner will spend a significant amount of time doing speed training. This can result in greater efficiency in removing lactate from the muscle blood flow and can help reduce the effects of muscle fatigue on performance.

5.3 Power

Power can be defined as the rate at which work is performed under a given set of conditions (work is the amount of force generated through a distance over time). In many sports power is often the single most important factor in achieving peak performance. However, optimum gains may only be achieved if strength and speed are developed together.

It is the emphasis on power that makes power training essential to sports which on first inspection would not appear to benefit from strength training. A games player will need more strength and power than a 1500 metre runner, although both require some strength and power training. A rugby forward needs more strength than a winger (eg to hold position in a scrum), however, a winger needs to be more powerful than a forward (eg to hand off the opposing players).

Power may not be produced without strength, therefore training programmes need to progress from strength to power development throughout the season. The aim of this variation is the production of peak power at the optimum time in the competitive season.

It is very difficult to classify each sport in terms of its exclusive energy requirements. For example, a swimmer will need power to push off the starting block but during the first length, speed demands take priority and at the turn the emphasis will be on power and flexibility. The performer will go flat out at the start but as the race continues the emphasis will change to speed endurance.

Consider the demands of your sport in terms of strength, speed and power requirements and the role each one plays to meet specific performance needs.

5.4 Effects of Strength Training

In order to design an appropriate and effective training programme, it is important to understand the physiological adaptations which result from strength training. Strength gains are usually accompanied by an increase in the diameter size of individual muscle fibres known as muscular **hypertrophy**. These changes are attributed to:

- increases in the number and size of myofibrils per muscle fibre (ie larger muscles)

- increases in amounts of contractile protein, particularly in the myosin filament (ie more forceful contraction)

- increases in amounts and strength of connective tendons and ligaments (ie greater stability)

- increased cross-sectional area of the muscle (ie generating more force)

- increased efficiency in muscle fibre recruitment (ie improvements in the nervous control of muscles).

It may help you to refer back to Sections 1.11–1.17 pages 23–35.

Each individual will have a predetermined strength potential due to genetic, age and sex differences. The relative proportions of muscle fibre types (pages 27–28) are particularly significant. To some extent muscle fibre types can be influenced by training. However, an individual with a greater percentage of fast twitch fibres will respond considerably better to power weight training than someone with a large percentage of slow twitch fibres – these performers may well respond better to aerobic muscular endurance. Effective use of this information can benefit both coach and performer (eg selecting team positions relative to individual strength or endurance, or adapting sessions to create overload of specific muscle type according to function).

5.5 Principles of Strength Training

Strength training programmes should be constructed on sound principles which apply to the development of strength and power just as much as any other aspect of fitness. The following principles are applicable to strength training:

- **Progressive overload** is achieved by increasing the intensity, duration and frequency of the exercise. This is most effectively developed when the muscle or group of muscles is overloaded by contracting against resistances exceeding those normally encountered. This forces the muscle to contract at or near maximum which stimulates the physiological adaptations that lead to increased muscular strength.

- **Specificity** – remember the response to training is specific. The strength programmes which are devised must reflect the specific requirements of the sport and the particular needs of the performer. To achieve the best results, the exercises must directly reflect the pattern and execution of the muscle movements involved in the sport.

- **Adaptation and reversibility**. The body needs time to adapt to the overload being applied in order for tissue repair and growth to occur. Conversely, much of the adaptation achieved from training is reversible over a period of time if training is not maintained. It is generally considered that one-third of the intensity of the original strength training programme is required to maintain the level of strength achieved. The programme should not only be progressive but also continuous, avoiding prolonged periods of absence from training.

TASK

Strength gains are most rapid over the initial stages of a programme which is why stronger individuals often show a slower initial improvement. Consider the consequences of using the same programme for an adolescent performer new to your sport and an experienced trained adult. Would you expect each to reach the same level by following identical programmes?

Carefully tailored, individual training programmes will be required for both performers. Progression will only be achieved if appropriate training loads are set for each performer.

5.6 Strength Training Programmes

Before devising a strength training programme, it is important to consider the following in relation to the specific needs of the individual:

- **General strength** of the whole muscular system which forms the foundations for all strength training programmes.

- **Specific strength** of the muscles directly related to a particular sport (eg arm muscles of shot putter, leg muscles of speed skater or downhill skier).

- **Monitoring** and recording progress is essential to ensure effective progression.

- **Variation** in training methods to meet the needs of the performer. It is necessary to understand each

method and its relative effectiveness to ensure success. The following list shows the various methods which will be described in detail later in the chapter:

- free weights

- multi-station weight machines

- body resistance exercises

- isometric training

- isokinetic training

- plyometrics (explosive power training)

- pulleys and springs.

Safety

Safety is of paramount importance and coaches and performers should be aware of the safety precautions required before commencing any form of strength training.

To ensure safety, the following guidelines should be considered:

- It is essential to warm up and cool down before and after strength training to prevent possible injury of muscle tissue and joints.

- The correct lifting technique (Figure 36) must be learned in order to maximise gains and limit injuries resulting from poor posture and body alignment.

The dead lift:

- Feet should be hip-width apart, toes just under the bar and turned out.
- Bend at the knees and hips, head up and eyes looking forward with your back in its normal erect posture (your back will feel slightly arched)
- Hold the bar just wider than your feet; check that shoulders are above hips and hips above knees (a – start).
- Never lift with your spine curved as this can cause serious problems (c – incorrect start)
- Lift by straightening legs and hips. The bar should travel in front of the shins, past the knees and finish mid-thighs (b – finish).
- Breathe in as you stand up straight, breathe out as you lower – never hold your breath.

This method of lifting is vital to avoid back injury.

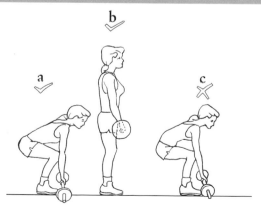

Figure 36: Principles of safe lifting – the dead lift

- **Resistance** (loading). It is dangerous to lift excessively heavy weights too soon. If the starting weight is kept low in the early stages, safe and efficient technique will be mastered more quickly.

- **The training area** should have adequate space and an even, firm, non-slip floor.

- **Equipment** should be soundly constructed, maintained and checked regularly.

- **Expert instruction and supervision.** When specialised equipment is used, qualified instruction must be sought.

Coaching children

Extensive weight training can cause damage to the developing body. Weight training with children requires a sensible, well informed approach, relevant coach expertise, sound technique and constant supervision.

5.7 Programme Content

Before a training programme can be designed, it is important to clarify a number of terms:

- **Repetition** (reps) is the number of times an exercise is performed without stopping.

- **Resistance** is the load which the muscle (or group of muscles) is required to move.

- **Repetition maximum** (RM) is the maximum load a muscle or group of muscles can lift a given number of times before fatiguing (eg a performer achieves the bench-press exercise ten times (and no more) in succession before fatiguing, then the weight used is the 10-RM load on that exercise).

Once the correct knowledge and equipment has been established, the details of the programme must then be considered and this means attention to:

- type of resistance

- frequency and duration

- speed

- rest.

Type of resistance

This depends on the type of strength being developed. Exercises which involve high repetitions and low resistances will improve the endurance qualities of the muscle, whereas low repetitions with high resistances develop pure strength.

A specific number of repetitions comprises one set (eg three sets of ten repetitions will be written as 3 x 10). It is not possible to state categorically which particular combination of sets and the maximum load will increase either muscular strength or muscular endurance more effectively. It depends on the individual and the specific requirements of the sport.

The maximum load that can be lifted once is known as the one repetition maximum (1-RM). The RM can be adjusted according to the programme (eg 3-RM represents the maximum load that can be lifted for three repetitions only). It has been found that significant strength gains can be achieved from programmes which consist of one to six repeats, with loads varying from 3-RM to 20-RM. These figures should be used as a broad guide only. Most programmes consist of between one and three sets and 5-RM to 10-RM loads.

Frequency and Duration

It is generally agreed that two to three exercise sessions per week produce significant gains in strength. This should prevent excessive stress on the performers by giving adequate recovery time between sessions. Each session should normally last from 45–90 minutes but this depends on the physical condition of the individual and the speed at which the exercise routines are carried out and the recovery time.

Speed

The optimum speed of a repetition will vary depending on the muscle group being used and the specific requirement of the sport. Faster repetitions are likely to produce a more dynamic kind of strength through nervous (neural) adaptations, while slower movements tend to produce adaptations within the muscle itself. When the speed of contraction is increased, it is important to maintain the full range of motion within the muscle(s) and the correct technique.

Rest between repetitions should be minimal to ensure overload (ie less than one second). Rest intervals between sets should be from 90–120 seconds depending on the intensity of the session. Bearing in mind the need for rest, it is advisable to exercise the larger, more powerful muscle groups before the smaller ones. This allows an effective overload in the larger muscles which will fatigue at a slower rate.

The exercises should be organised in a specific sequence to avoid using the same muscle group twice in a row (eg back exercise, arms, legs, abdominals in rotation). After a session of heavy weight lifting using a particular muscle group, the specific group will require a period of rest to help promote adaptation to training and replenish depleted energy stores.

5.8 Types of Programme

There are several types of programme that can be performed when using free weights or multi-station weight machines. Three of these methods include:

- weights circuit training
- progressive resistance training
- pyramid training.

Weights Circuit Training Method

The performer's 10-RM must first be established (the maximum load that can be lifted ten times without a break). A sensible sequence of exercises is chosen so that muscle groups are exercised in a specific order. This ensures that each group has an adequate recovery period. A set of 10 repetitions is performed at the 10-RM on each exercise, with 90–120 seconds recovery time between each exercise. Once all the exercises have been performed, the sequence is repeated two or three times depending on the individual's fitness level.

Progressive Resistance Method

The performer's 10-RM must first be established. On each exercise the performer will carry out three sets of ten repetitions, with a recovery period of 90–120 seconds.

The target is to complete three sets of ten repetitions at 100% of 10-RM load. However, it is more likely that the performer will manage all ten repetitions during the first set, fewer (eg eight) during the second set and possibly only six or seven during the third set.

In time (ie training three times a week for a number of weeks), the performer will be able to complete all three sets of ten repetitions at that load. After this, the performers's new 10-RM should be assessed and used during subsequent training. In this way, progressive overload is maintained.

Pyramid Method

Establish the 2-RM. The programme involves increasing the load while decreasing the number of repetitions. It is a very advanced method of training and should not be attempted without expert instruction.

> For example, if the 2-RM is 25 kg:
>
> Set 1 = six reps at 5kg
> Set 2 = five reps at 10kg
> Set 3 = four reps at 15kg
> Set 4 = three reps at 20kg
> Set 5 = two reps at 25kg.

The increase in load between repeats can be between 2.5–5kg depending on the individual performer (recovery period of 90–120 seconds between sets). As soon as the performer can achieve five repetitions in the final set, the loads in every set should be increased.

5.9 Methods of Strength/Power Training

Strength and power training can cause debilitating injuries if the exercises are not correctly performed. To avoid such injuries and optimise training benefits, there should be a sensible progression from the fundamental body weight exercises to the more advanced multi-gym training, free weights and the specialised plyometric power training exercises.

The following examples of strength training methods reflect this line of progression:

- body resistance exercises
- body resistance exercises with a partner
- body resistance exercises using simple equipment
- multi-station weight machines
- free weights
- isometric training
- isokinetic training
- plyometrics
- speed training.

Body Resistance Exercises

Body weight exercises provide an ideal first stage in the development of speed and power. This method of training offers the opportunity to learn basic technique and build a firm foundation for general strength. It can take place almost anywhere (eg on a games field, athletics track or in a gymnasium). As performers are using their own body weight, incorrect technique is less likely to result in injury. It is especially recommended for:

- relatively untrained individuals
- those below the age of 18 years when the bones and muscles are still developing and may not be strong enough to undertake strenuous weight training.

The intensity of training can be easily increased by adapting the exercises (eg change of body position, use of partners) or by using simple equipment or apparatus.

TASK

You may wish to work practically through the following exercises (press-up to press behind neck) and assess the possible benefits to your sport.

Individual Body Resistance Exercises

The following sets of exercises demonstrate how variation and differences in resistance can be introduced into simple exercises:

Press-up

- Body part: chest, back of upper arm, front shoulder.
- Muscles: pectorals, triceps, anterior deltoid.

Start facing ground, with hands shoulder width apart and knees and feet on floor. Straighten arms, raising chest off floor. Reverse action to lower chest to floor again. Keep head in line with spine.

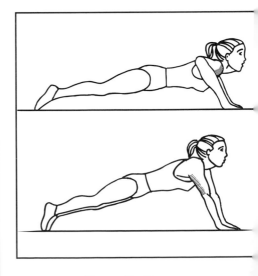

Figure 37: Press-up

Progression:

- Move elbows close to body to increase intensity in back of upper arm (triceps).

- Move elbows out to side to increase tension on chest muscles (pectorals).

- Extend legs back so feet rest on floor to increase intensity of all muscle groups involved.

- Increase variety of exercises (eg finger tip press-up, press-up clapping hands, press-up feet raised and one arm press-up).

Abdominal crunch

- **Body part**: abdominals (upper, lower, side).

- **Muscles**: rectus abdominis, transverse abdominis, external/internal obliques.

Lie on floor mat, with legs bent and hands on knees. With chin on chest, curl up pushing lower back into mat. Lower to start position.

NB   It is important to note that if sit ups are performed with the feet anchored, then the emphasis will be on working the hip flexors and not the abdominal muscles.

Progression:

- Cross arms in front of chest.

- Fully extend arms out to the sides (crucifix).

Squat thrust

- **Body part**: buttocks, front and back thigh, calves.

- **Muscles**: gluteals, quadriceps, hamstring, gastrocnemius, soleus (shoulder muscles (deltoids) act as fixators).

Place hands in front, shoulder width apart with legs extended behind and feet on floor. By lifting feet off floor, bring knees in towards chest. Reverse to start position by thrusting legs behind.

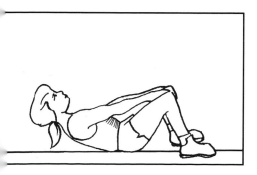

Figure 38: Abdominal crunch

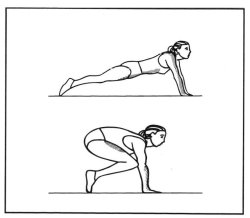

Figure 39: Squat thrust

Progression:

- Standing squat. From upright position, bend from hips to lower knees to 90° angle. Keeping back straight and head up, return to standing.

- Squat jump. Standing movement from squat is extended to jump.

It is advantageous to vary the exercises regularly to reduce boredom and the risk of injury. Coaches should always ensure all performers carry out the movements correctly.

Body Resistance Exercises with a Partner

The body weight exercises mainly utilise isotonic contractions and many of them can be used as part of a circuit training programme. It is possible to use some safe partner work in developing strength and these might include more isometric contractions where a muscle group is working without causing movement around a joint.

Separate Wrists
Partners attempt to separate wrists.

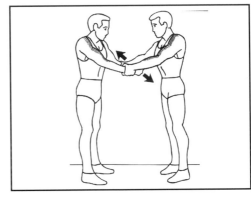

Figure 40: Separate wrists

Separate Legs
Partners try to push legs apart.

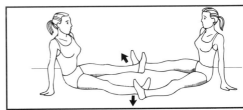

Figure 41: Separate legs

Separate Hands
Partners attempt to clap hands overhead.

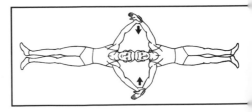

Figure 42: Separate hands

Upright Stand

Partners try to stand alternately.

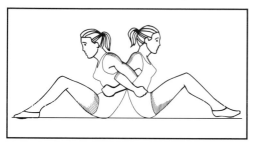

Figure 43: Upright stand

Body Resistance Exercises Using Simple Equipment

The following activities make use of gymnasium apparatus but utilise body weight as the resistance.

Using a Beam or High Bar

Raise knees to chest. Remember to keep the back straight and only use the hip flexors (do not hyper-flex the spine).

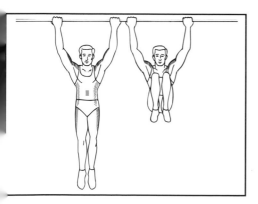

Figure 44: Using a beam or high bar

Using Parallel Bars

Lowering arms to 90° at elbow.

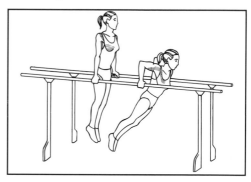

Figure 45: Using parallel bars

Multi-station Weight Machines

The universal or multi-gym provides a wide range of exercises while offering some degree of assistance with the learning of new techniques. There are also many single-unit exercise stations which have been developed. Their design allows a quick and easy change of resistance. Pulleys and springs offer the facility to change the angle of force or vary resistances. However, the fixator muscles are not fully trained which limits the total strength gains in comparison to free weight methods.

A basic multi-gym programme may include the following exercises:
Leg press, bench press and leg curl (described over the page).

Leg Press

- **Body part**: front thigh, calves.
- **Muscles**: quadriceps, gastrocnemius.

Sit with back firmly against seat; angle at knee joint should be 90°. Holding seat rails, press feet firmly against pedals and extend legs. Avoid over-extending knee joint. Note maximum resistance moved. Slowly return weight stack to start position.

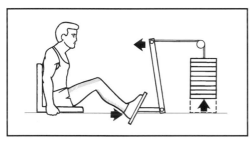

Figure 46: Leg press

Bench Press

- **Body part**: chest, back of upper arm, front shoulder.
- **Muscles**: pectorals, triceps, anterior deltoid.

Place bench approximately two inches from weight stack. Lie face up on bench with head nearest apparatus and feet placed flat on floor. Grip bars (one and a half shoulder width apart). Leading with knuckles, extend arms to raise weights but avoid over-extension of elbow joint. Leading with elbows, lower stack to start position.

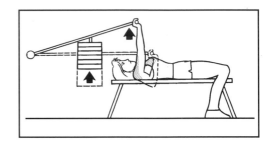

Figure 47: Bench press

Leg Curl

- **Body part**: back of thigh, calves.
- **Muscles**: hamstring, gastrocnemius.

Lie face down with knees resting on edge of bench. Flex knees to bring heels towards buttocks as far as possible. Return under control but do not lock out knees. Remember to keep knees slightly bent and head in line with spine.

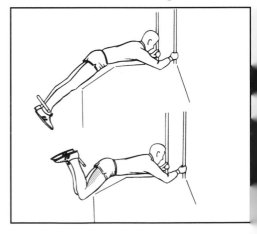

Figure 48: Leg curl

Free Weights

Performers must be strong in many movements and this will obviously vary according to the sport. Many of these movements rely on the stabiliser muscles (Section 1.14 page 30) to maintain the correct position. The versatility of free weights enables the use of specific exercises reflecting those actions commonly used in a specific sport, resulting in strength gains throughout the whole range of movement. To avoid injury, it is very important to use the correct techniques and a spotter (someone to help you if any difficulties arise during the exercise). A few exercises using free weights are described.

Clean (Power Clean)

- **Body part:** lower back, front/back thigh, calves, shoulder, front upper arm.

- **Muscles:** erector spinae, quadriceps, hamstring, gastrocnemius, soleus, deltoids, biceps.

Stand with shins touching bar, feet hip width apart, toes turned slightly outwards. Grip bar, hands shoulder-width apart, assume position in diagram, with flat solid back. Arms should remain straight, eyes looking straight ahead, shoulders higher than hips. Lift bar by extending legs and back. Keep arms straight. Extend body upwards by raising onto toes then shrugging shoulders, rotate wrists to receive bar onto front of shoulders, bend at knees to cushion weight. To return bar to floor, lower to thighs and then to floor. Breathe in for lift and out as bar is lowered.

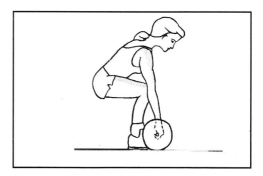

Figure 49: Clean

Straight Arm Pullover

- **Body part**: chest, shoulder, back of upper arm.
- **Muscles**: pectorals, deltoid, triceps.

This exercise requires either two helpers or two support racks on which to place bar. Lie on bench, face up with feet resting firmly on ground and turned slightly outwards, knees bent at right angles. Take weight on outstretched arms, above upper chest, with palms under and supporting bar. Lower bar under control to chest leading with elbow. Breathe in when lowering bar and out as arms extend.

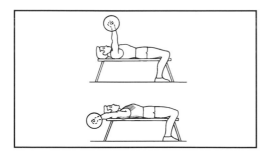

Figure 50: Straight arm pullover

Front Squat

- **Body part**: lower back, buttocks, front thigh, calves.
- **Muscles**: erector spinae, gluteals, quadriceps, gastrocnemius.

Rest bar across upper chest, feet hip-width apart. Take an undergrip on bar, thumbs forward. Hold head up, look straight ahead, keeping back straight. Lower hips and bar by bending from hips and knees. Keep back flat, control downward movement, then powerfully lift weight back to starting position. Straighten legs and press hips forward under bar to maintain a strong lifting position. Breathe in before starting lift and out as bar is raised.

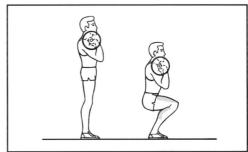

Figure 51: Front squat

Arm Curl

- **Body part**: front of upper arm, forearm.
- **Muscles**: biceps, brachialis.

Stand with feet comfortably apart. Grip bar with undergrasp just wider than shoulder-width. Hold bar across upper part of thighs, arms fully extended. Slowly flexing arms, raise bar to chest. Keep head up and back straight throughout. Reverse action to lower bar, keeping the body trunk still. Breathe in when lifting bar and out when lowering it.

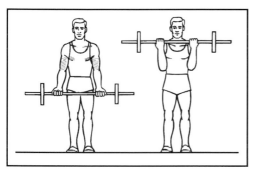

Figure 52: Arm curl

Calf Raise

- **Body part**: calves.

- **Muscles**: gastrocnemius, soleus.

Rest bar on trapezius muscles of shoulder with feet slightly wider than hip-width apart. Raise heels as high as possible and lower them again under control. Breathe in when raising body and out when lowering.

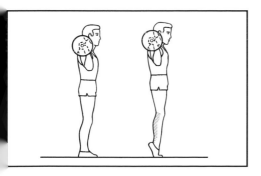

Figure 53: Calf raise

Press Behind Neck

- **Body part**: shoulder, upper back, back of upper arm.

- **Muscles**: deltoids, trapezius, triceps.

Rest bar on trapezius muscle of shoulder with feet slightly more than hip-width apart and hands slightly more than shoulder-width apart. Press bar overhead by extending arms leading with knuckles. Do not lock out elbow joint. Lower back to shoulders. Breathe in as bar is pressed up and out as it is lowered.

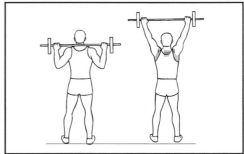

Figure 54: Press behind neck

When you consider strength training for children, it is important to:

- avoid weights which overload growing bones because doing so may damage the epiphyses
- use only light weights, or no weights at all, until after growth spurts
- use the resistance caused by the child's own body to promote sufficient strength gains
- develop muscular endurance by light resistances and a high number of repetitions (eg circuits).

At all stages, it is most important to emphasise the learning of good techniques in carrying out exercises. Coaches should know the techniques before trying to teach them, ensuring safety and allowing for the most benefit to be gained from the exercise.

Isometric Training

Isometrics involve muscular contractions performed against an immovable resistance or load. Best results are obtained if the tension generated by the muscle is at or near maximum. It is advisable to train a maximum of three times a week in order to allow sufficient time to recover.

Strength development in isometric training will be greatest at the joint angle at which the exercise is performed (eg if the leg is being trained with the knee flexed at right angles, the limb becomes stronger when flexed at that angle). If strength is required over the full range of movement, then exercises must be performed at several different angles.

Many sports require isometric strength and endurance (eg wrestling, where strength is required to resist or reposition the opponent, gymnastics where the gymnast is required to balance and sustain certain body positions).

The correct breathing technique is very important during isometric training, as a respiratory effort is made with the epiglottis closed so air cannot escape. If the performer does not exhale while performing the isometric contraction, blood pressure rises above normal levels which is potentially very dangerous and in extreme cases can be fatal.

Gymnasts will often rely on isometric muscle action to maintain position in a particular extreme movement (eg holding the crucifix position on the rings). However, gymnasts must also prepare the fixator muscles which assist in stabilising the joint (eg shoulder and upper back muscles) to avoid muscle tear and potential dislocation.

Analyse the movements in your sport that may benefit from isometric training. Explain how you can ensure the fixator muscles are equally trained.

Isokinetic Training

Isokinetic training uses specialised machines (eg Cybex machines) and weight training apparatus to provide a resistance equal to the force being applied by the performer throughout the full range of movement. This results in equal strength gains which is a valuable training factor, since in most sports muscular force is applied during movement at various speeds.

A limb speed which is close to that used in a particular sport (eg the arm action of front crawl) can be pre-set using specialised machines. These machines allow the performer to exert optimal force and velocity at each point throughout the entire range of the movement. Any effort encounters an opposing force relative to the force being applied.

Theoretically, isokinetic training should make it possible to activate the largest number of motor units and consistently overload muscles to achieve maximum force at every point in the range of motion, even at relatively weaker joint angles.

Plyometrics

This method of training is a very effective means of power training and can be used in nearly all sports. When people attempt a vertical jump, no matter how bent their legs at the start, they will dip immediately before jumping. This dip causes a plyometric loading on the thigh muscles and stimulates a greater jump. Plyometric training takes advantage of this process, involving forceful action of muscle groups immediately after a loading which causes the muscle to stretch slightly (eg in bounding, squats, split squat).

Plyometrics is an advanced training technique using many exercises to develop power in different muscle groups. Expert instruction is vital before initiating any programme involving such techniques, due to the danger of damaging connective muscle tissue and growth plates. Coaches must take great care when working with young performers and plyometrics.

Speed Training

When considering speed work, it is important for the coach or performer to decide which component of speed should be trained (eg sprint swimmers may want to train on maximum speed rather than speed endurance).

Reaction speed drills

A reaction is a bodily response to an external stimulus. For example, an athlete responds to a starting gun by moving from the starting blocks as quickly as possible.

There are many factors (psychological and physiological) which influence reaction time and the initiation of movement. Figure 55 shows how the nervous system responds to an external factor. Usually response time can be improved with practise by improving movement time, provided the practice situation simulates the actual sport.

Developing anticipation is an important factor. Some top performers perform poorly on pure reaction tests but have such well developed anticipation that their results in a game situation are outstanding.

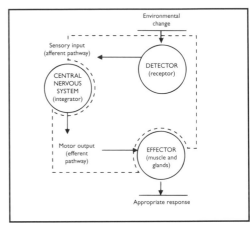

Figure 55: Response of nervous system to an external factor (eg starting gun)

There is a whole range of possible *reaction time* drills[1]. The following provide a guide which can be adapted for specific sports:

- Work in pairs (A and B). Partner B stands directly behind A. With accurate feeding of height and distance to provide just the right challenge, B throws a tennis ball forward over A's shoulder. On first sight of the ball, A runs forward to make a catch before the second bounce.

- Work in pairs (A and B). Partner A stands in ready position, B stands behind A's back holding a tennis ball at head height. B drops the tennis ball and on hearing the ball bounce on the floor, A turns to catch the ball before it bounces a second time. For progression, the difficulty can be

1   These are often referred to as *reaction time drills* but are actually *movement time drills*.

increased by dropping the ball from shoulder height, hip height or knee height. It is effective to do a set number of repetitions at each height and produce a small schedule.

- Work in threes (A, B and C). Stand five metres apart, each holding a tennis ball. A faces B with a distance of five metres between them. B throws ball to A who returns it to B, then A runs to a point opposite C who throws the ball to A who returns it to C. A then runs back in front of B. This small pressure practice continues for a set time interval of 60 seconds.

TASK

Reaction speed is important in a 100m sprint race lasting for less than ten seconds. Olympic sprinter Linford Christie trains to respond quickly to the starter's gun. In skiing and canoe slalom competitions, rapid reaction is needed to change direction, in combat sports (karate and fencing) quick responses are also vital.

You may find it useful to identify where fast response demands occur in your sport.

Running Speed Drills

Since the propulsive force is created by the extension of the driving leg, this action should receive particular attention when training for sprinting. Coaches must remember that any training programme to improve this quality needs to be supplemented by carefully structured strength and flexibility work. Muscle groups (eg the quadriceps, gluteals and gastrocnemius) need to be strengthened so they can contract more powerfully. Co-ordination between the contracting (prime mover) and relaxing (antagonist) muscle groups must be developed.

Training for speed work helps the performer to withstand the build-up of high levels of hydrogen ions associated with lactate in the muscles (which can contribute to fatigue; see page 87) and increases the ability to remove both hydrogen ions and lactate. The following examples can be used as guidelines when designing a particular training programme:

Running on the spot

Work in pairs, facing each other, one metre apart. Run on the spot, knees high with exaggerated arm movements. Two or three sets of a given drill should be performed with rest intervals appropriate for the level of fitness.

One set of this drill might be:

- half speed for 20–30 seconds, with a 60 second walk recovery
- three-quarter speed for 20–30 seconds with a 60 second walk recovery
- seven-eight speed for 10–15 seconds with a 60 second walk recovery.
- half speed for 20–30 seconds, with a 60 second walk recovery
- three-quarter speed for 20–30 seconds with a 60 second walk recovery
- seven-eight speed for 10–15 seconds with a 60 second walk recovery.

Speed endurance exercises

These exercises can be performed in sets (normally at less than maximum speed) with the recovery periods adapted to suit the performer's fitness level (eg squat jumping, squat thrust, abdominal curl and press ups). Speed endurance is frequently used in running events and by games players and is used in the following three modes:

- **Acceleration sprints.** These gradually increase from a rolling start to jogging, to striding out to maximum pace. The recovery period at the end of each sequence should be a 30–50 second walk or jog. This exercise is particularly useful for emphasising and maintaining the technical component of the sprinting action as speed increases.

- **Hollow sprints.** These use brief sprints interrupted by a period of recovery in the form of light running or jogging (eg accelerate for 30–50 metres, jog 10–30 metres, accelerate again for 30–50 metres, then walk for 100–150 metres as the recovery phase). This form of training is appropriate to games players, as it offers a variation in speed and tempo within each sequence.

- **Repetition sprints.** This involves running fixed distances at constant speed (75–100% of maximum speed) with recovery periods of sufficient length to allow the performer to maintain form and the required degree of quality. Games players could do sets of 20–70 metre sprints with jog recovery.

Other types of sprint training include:

- **sprint-assisted** training which includes downhill running, towing and treadmill running, which all assist in increasing stride frequency
- **sprint-resisted** training which includes uphill running, weighted clothing and running in sand which increases strength, aerobic and muscular endurance.

5.10 Cyclical Year-round Strength Training Programme

With all forms of training, there is a definite need for long-term planning, as any physiological adaptations which take place will be the result of training during an extended period. During this programme there are three distinct areas of work:

1 General strength

2 Specific strength

3 Competition strength.

The emphasis on each will depend on the specific sport and its competition calendar. The development of both general and specific strength are prerequisites to competition based strength. Competition strength involves whole technique exercises simulating the type and nature of the muscular work occurring in competition.

Naturally there are considerable variations between sports but most have a competitive season of a certain length which allows a cyclical year-round programme to be planned. This can be based on the following defined periods: off-season period, pre-season period, competition period.

Off-season Period

During the off-season period (recovery and rest), there should be a gradual decrease in all forms of training to a point of complete rest. This period should, however, be tailored to an individual performer's need. For example, some performers prefer to maintain lighter forms of activity rather than complete rest (eg distance swimmers).

Pre-season Period

There are usually two phases within the pre-season period:

- **Preparation phase** (conditioning) where general strength is developed as a basis for specialised strength.

- **Training phase** (building strength) where specialised strength is developed to meet the demands of the sport.

Competition Period

During the competition period (because of the reversibility of training effects), the approach should be to maintain levels of specialised strength while incorporating competition based exercises which are closely related to the techniques of the sport. This period generally has two phases:

- **Early competitive phase** (developing power) where specialised and competition-based strength is developed.

- **Major competitive phase** (maintaining power) where the specialised and competitive-based strength developed in the previous phase are maintained.

5.11 Tests of Strength, Speed and Power

In order to achieve progression, the effects of any training programme must be carefully monitored and adapted accordingly. Strength, speed and power tests provide useful feedback to the performer and will help maintain motivation out of competition season. The following examples offer simple but nonetheless accurate tests covering all three areas of strength training.

Strength

Repetition maximums (eg 1-RM = the total weight lifted in one repetition prior to muscle overload) are often used. The 1-RM method requires a good standard of weightlifting skill and experience, therefore tests should only be administered if a good level of lifting skill is reached. Such tests should be carried out on a regular basis (eg early part of a training phase and latter part of a training phase), in similar conditions ensuring

maintenance of good technique. The exercise used ideally should reflect the specific sport.

Speed

Sprint tests are ideal and very versatile when it comes to testing speed. They also represent more closely many of the demands placed on performers during competition (eg racket ball players and field athletes). Both reaction and running time can be assessed by adapting the tests.

Power

Lower body power can be tested by use of the sergeant jump for height (Figure 56). The performer stands with feet shoulder-width apart, heels on the ground about 20–30 cms from a wall. Having previously dipped fingers in chalk, the performer jumps up and makes a finger mark at the highest possible point.

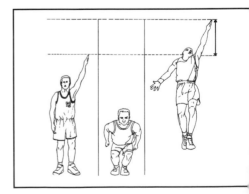

Figure 56: Example of the sergeant jump used to test power

TASK

To gain maximum benefit, power tests should be chosen to reflect the specific sport (eg testing a boxer for lower body power is obviously inappropriate, when their upper body punch power is of greater importance; cyclists, however, need a greater reliance on leg power).

Consider the important aspects of your sport and which tests would be most beneficial.

5.12 Summary

All sporting activities will require some degree of strength; which type will obviously relate to the specific sport. If training is to be successful, exercises must directly relate to the pattern and execution of those movements required during competition. Any training programme must take into account the type of strength, speed or power needed, the muscle groups involved and the facilities available. An understanding of the role that strength, speed and power plays in relation to overall performance is vital in optimising gains during training and competition.

Further reading to supplement this knowledge can be found in the following texts:

Baechle, TR and Earle, RW (2000) **Essentials of strength training and conditioning**. Champaign IL, Human Kinetics. ISBN 0 736000 89 5

Chu, D A (1998) **Jumping into plyometrics.** Champaign IL, Human Kinetics. ISBN 0 880118 46 6

*Davies, J (1996) **Fitness for games players.** Leeds, National Coaching Foundation. ISBN 0 947850 10 4

* Available from **Coachwise 1st4sport** (tel 0113-201 5555 or visit www.1st4sport.com).

Fleck, SJ and Kraemer, WJ (1997) **Designing resistance training programs**. Champaign IL, Hman Kinetics. ISBN 0 873225 08 2

Komi, P V (1991) **Strength and power in sport**. Oxford, Blackwell Scientific. ISBN 0 632 03806 3

Norris, C (2001) **Weight training principles and practice.** London, A & C Black. ISBN 0 713637 71 4

Paish, W (1991) **Training for peak performance.** London, A & C Black. ISBN 0 713634 04 9

*Wilkinson, D and Moore, P (1995) **A guide to field based fitness testing**. Leeds, National Coaching Foundation. ISBN 0 947850 55 4

*   Complimentary with the **sports coach UK** Performance Coach Workshop *Field Based Fitness Testing* or available from **Coachwise 1st4sport** (tel 0113-201 5555 or visit www.1st4sport.com).

TASK

The following tasks will help you to relate the knowledge provided in this chapter to a practical coaching situation. A firm foundation based on the principles of training will ensure a training programme achieves its goals and ensures the performer is participating at maximum potential.

1   Devise a weight training circuit (with appropriate supervision) to include all the major muscle groups. Determine your 3-RM by lifting progressively heavier weights until you achieve overload of the muscle. Notice the differences in weights achieved by various muscle groups. Would all performers of the same level but different sports achieve similar results? How can individual differences be considered in a group situation?

2   How would you adapt a training session to train the slow twitch and fast twitch fibres respectively? Does strength, speed and power training have to be specific to a sport? In what way can development of these factors assist within your particular sport?

CHAPTER SIX:
Flexibility

6.0 Introduction

While most coaches and performers recognise the importance of endurance, strength, power and speed, the role of **flexibility** is often neglected. A balanced fitness programme incorporating all the elements of total fitness is essential to achieve maximum gains.

Flexibility is the only aspect of fitness with which everyone is born but even between babies and very young children, individual differences in flexibility exist. The movement habits adopted in early life greatly influence how much flexibility is retained in later years.

Flexibility training should be specific and safe, especially with children as their flexible bodies are more vulnerable to injury.

6.1 What is It?

Flexibility is defined as the range of movement around a joint (eg the knee) or a series of joints (eg the spinal column). It results from the stretching of muscles and connective tissues around the joints and not from the looseness of the capsule or ligaments.

With all components of fitness (ie endurance, strength and speed), performers need a planned programme to gain or maintain flexibility. To achieve maximum gains, the ideal flexibility training for most sports would be an hour a day. However, the requirement for each sport will vary along with available training time.

TASK

At this point it may be of value to refer to Section 1.7 page 12 to recap on the structure and function of the synovial joint. Think how the muscle groups work in pairs (eg as the front thigh muscle (quadriceps) contracts, the back of the thigh (hamstrings) oppose the movement which then restricts movement at the knee joint). Flexibility exercises that gently stretch the fibrous tissues of these muscles around the knee encourage them to lengthen and thus reduce resistance at the knee joint. This increases the availability of synovial fluid to the knee, thus providing lubrication. As muscles naturally tighten and become shorter with training, it is essential they are stretched.

Choose one common movement in your sport (eg a turn or a throw) and identify flexibility exercises which can be used to prepare the body for action.

6.2 Stretching Routines

It is important at this stage to distinguish between stretching as part of flexibility training and stretching in a warm-up/cool-down.

The main aim of:

- **flexibility training** is to improve the current range of movement about the joints during a specific session

- **warm-up stretching** is to prepare the performer before activity (this maintains but will not improve flexibility)

- **cool-down stretching** is to relax and reduce muscle soreness following activity (this maintains but will not improve flexibility).

6.3 Importance of Flexibility

The importance of flexibility has long been recognised. It may help to:

- **prevent injury** by developing the soft tissue of the muscle in reducing resistance to movement and increasing protection from damage[1]

- **improve performance** by using the full range of motion around a given joint.

An element of flexibility is important for all sports – however in certain sports, the importance of developing flexibility is obvious (eg gymnastics). Most sports do not require such extreme ranges of movement as gymnastics. It is important to develop flexibility to a level that allows the optimal performance of specific skills. For example, in a sliding tackle in soccer, the adductor muscles of the thigh can be protected from injury by good static flexibility.

There is a tendency to think of flexibility in association with one joint at a time but this is quite misleading. If a performer's movement is restricted because of a lack of flexibility (eg in the hamstrings), then a compensatory movement in the lumbar spine may give the desired result but may also be detrimental in the long-term (or even in the short-term). Therefore, balanced flexibility is needed, so that all areas of the body can be optimally responsive while maintaining the skilled movement. Even if a particular sport requires some joints to be more flexible than others, it is important to keep a balanced programme of training to avoid relying on compensatory movements. This may seem like an argument against specificity of training and to some extent

---

1 Although there is no direct evidence to support the benefits of flexibility, it is generally agreed that stretching may help to reduce the likelihood of injury.

it is; the main aim should be to move all areas of restricted movements towards their optimal level of functional flexibility.

6.4 Factors Affecting Flexibility

The full potential range of movement possible at any given joint or series of joints will be limited by the following factors:

- **Shape and structure of the bone and joint**
  The type of joint will obviously dictate the movement possible. For example, the knee is a hinge joint that only allows movement in one plane. Therefore, any exercise that attempts to rotate the joint can lead to serious injury. The structure of a joint must be considered when designing a safe and effective programme.

- **Condition of the muscles and ligaments**
  The condition of the muscles and ligaments plays a major role in determining the range of movement of a joint. Stretching the elastic tissue in the muscle before contraction will limit resistance to movement and protect the joint from damage. An understanding of the structure of muscles and their attachments will further enhance safe and effective performance (Section 1.12 page 25).

- **Temperature of the body and muscles**
  Increases in local muscle temperature actively promote increased mobility as the connective tissue, ligaments and tendons become more pliable. Additionally, the synovial fluid becomes less dense and resistance to movement decreases. The range of movement allowed by the muscle decreases as it cools. This is due to the slowing down of the chemical reactions involved in contraction and the reduced elasticity of the muscle. Research has shown increases in muscle force production of 10–15% for every 1°C rise in muscle temperature.

- **Age and sex of the performer**
  General flexibility will decrease with age but stretching can help delay the shortening of the muscles and connective tissues associated with ageing. The optimum range for improvement is during childhood when greater calcification of cartilage occurs and the surrounding tissues of the joint promote elasticity and ease of movement. It has been shown that women are generally more flexible than men. This may be due to anatomical differences as the flexibility variation is greater after puberty.

6.5 Types of Flexibility

There are two main types of flexibility:

- **Static** which is a measure of the extent to which a joint may be moved slowly and held (eg lowering yourself slowly to perform the splits).

- **Dynamic** which is a measure of the range of movement around a joint through active muscular contraction (eg jumping in the air while drawing the legs apart to perform the splits).

TASK

The significance of these limiting effects cannot be taken for granted. Gymnasts require a great deal of flexibility (eg hip abduction on the asymmetric bars) but the structural differences imposed by such joints will not improve with training. Hypermobility (hyperextension of a joint, often called double-jointedness) resulting from laxity of the ligaments and capsules is an advantage in some sports. However, problems occur through over extension once the joint passes outside its normal range of activity, when it might become unstable and lead to injury or dislocation (eg shoulder joint).

Think of the activities in your sport that require joint stability and those that benefit from increased mobility.

6.6 Methods of Stretching

Stretching is the method used to increase flexibility. There are three main types of stretching:

- Static

- Ballistic

- Proprioceptive neuromuscular facilitation (PNF).

Static Stretching

Static stretching is also known as slow or passive stretching. The antagonist muscle is placed in a position of maximum stretch. The sensory endings within the muscle spindles are stretched which result in sensory impulses being sent to the brain. This triggers a reflex contraction resisting the stretch known as the **stretch reflex**. By holding the stretch for 10–15 seconds, desensitisation of the stretch reflex occurs, allowing the muscle to be stretched without causing damage to the fibres or connective tissues.

Slow static stretching is achieved by:

- ensuring the muscle is thoroughly warm first

- staying relaxed and unhurried

- pulling the target muscle slowly towards its limit

- holding the stretch for 10–15 seconds

- increasing the stretch to new limits
- holding for 10–15 seconds then relaxing and repeating.

Ballistic Stretching

Ballistic stretching is often called fast, active or bouncing stretching. It involves the repetitive contraction of the agonistic muscle to give quick stretches to the antagonistic muscle. This is achieved by a series of bouncing or jerking movements which increase momentum in the body parts and drive the joint beyond its current range of movement.

These actions can be dangerous as the forces generated by jerks and bounces often exceed the extensibility limits of the tissues. Physical damage due to microscopic tearing of the muscle fibres may occur, causing scar tissue to form resulting in muscle soreness and loss of muscle elasticity. **Coaches should educate their performers to avoid the use of ballistic stretching.** The development of flexibility through static stretching is a gradual process and the performer must realise that bouncing will not accelerate flexibility gains.

Proprioceptive Neuromuscular Facilitation (PNF)

It must be stressed that this is an advanced form of stretching which is potentially dangerous. Expert instruction is vital to avoid damage to the muscles, connective tissue and their attachments. PNF normally requires either the coach to work with the performer or performers to work with each other in flexibility training.

NB Specific training is required before any coach attempts to incorporate PNF within a specific programme. Poor instruction could result in permanent damage to the performer.

TASK

Inappropriate and potentially dangerous flexibility exercises can be avoided by applying your knowledge of the structure and function of the body. For example, when performing a sitting groin stretch, you should not initiate the movement forward from the head and shoulders. This will round the shoulders and put pressure on lower back (Figure 57 shows both the correct and incorrect ways of performing this stretch). Coaches must ensure the flexibility exercises they use are appropriate to the muscle and joint, and specific to the sport to ensure maximum gains in performance and to avoid injury.

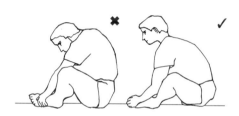

Figure 57: Incorrect and correct sitting groin stretch

What type of stretching do you use in your sport ?

6.7 Guidelines for Stretching

Like any other component of fitness, stretching programmes should reflect the principles of training (Section 5.5 page 119) which include the following:

- **Frequency**. Ideally stretching exercises should be carried out every day for an hour to maximise development. The performer must realise that gains in flexibility come gradually and will decline if stretching is not regularly maintained. However, once attained the gains are fairly persistent and can last up to a month after regular training.

- **Intensity**. Performers should passively stretch muscles to the point of slight discomfort, **not** pain. The stretch should be slow and controlled, concentrating on correct body alignment and muscle relaxation.

- **Time or duration**. The stretch should be held long enough for the stretch reflex to be desensitised (10–15 secs). Research suggests 30 seconds is most suitable to increase flexibility. Each stretch should be performed three or four times within a stretching routine.

6.8 Flexibility Exercises

There are numerous flexibility exercises designed for sports in general. It is important to adopt a whole body approach when designing a programme to maintain a balance. Developmental stretches (held for at least 30 seconds) aim to increase the range of movement at a joint and therefore should be appropriate to the sport. Maintenance stretches (held for 10–15 seconds) are important to sustain general flexibility and are of particular importance during warm-up and cool-down periods.

The following examples are given to show a balanced selection of stretches of the major muscle groups which can be used as a basis for a more detailed programme relative to the performer's needs.

TASK

You may find it useful to work through the following stretches (neck stretch to cat stretch) practically, concentrating on good technique and feeling the point of tension.

Neck Stretch

Stand in a balanced and comfortable position. Slowly move chin down towards top of chest, hold position, then push chin up and forwards. Hold for 30 seconds. Keep back straight. Do not circle head around neck as this can cause damage to the spine.

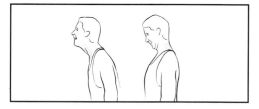

Figure 58: Neck stretch

Shoulder, Forearms Stretch

Link fingers together, palms turned outward. Extend arms out in front at shoulder height until slight discomfort is felt in shoulders, middle of upper back, arms, hands, fingers and wrist. Hold for 30 seconds. Slowly return to starting position. Repeat.

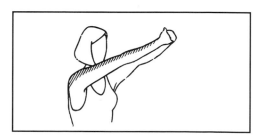

Figure 59: Shoulder, forearms stretch

Back of Upper Arm, Shoulder Stretch

Hold elbow of right arm with left hand, pull elbow behind head as shown, until slight discomfort is felt in back of upper arm and top of shoulders. Hold for 30 seconds. Slowly return to starting position. Repeat with left arm.

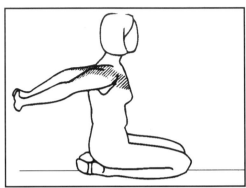

Figure 61: Chest stretch

Side Stretch

Stand with feet shoulder width apart, toes pointing forward. With right arm extended above head, bend sideways to left from hip; use left hand as support, until slight discomfort is felt down right side of body. Hold for 30 seconds. Slowly return to starting point. Repeat on opposite side.

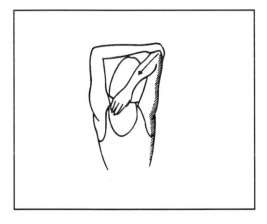

Figure 60: Back of upper arm, shoulder stretch

Chest Stretch

Sit with back to the wall, arm's length away. Link fingers of both hands together, with arms outstretched behind back. Pull arms up, brushing hands up wall until slight discomfort is felt in chest, shoulders and upper arms. Hold for 30 seconds. Slowly return to starting point. Repeat. Keep back straight, do not lean forward.

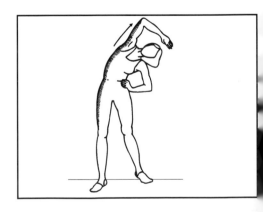

Figure 62: Side stretch

Quadriceps and Ankle Stretch

Lie on left side, rest head in palm of left hand. Gently pull ankle of right leg towards right hip until slight discomfort is felt. Hold for 30 seconds. Slowly return to starting position. Repeat. Turn onto right side and repeat with opposite leg.

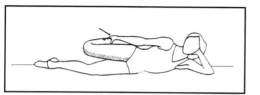

Figure 63: Quadriceps and ankle stretch

Hamstring Stretch

Lie on floor, back straight, raise left leg as shown in Figure 61. Keep right foot on floor with knee bent. Hold onto left leg near ankle and gently pull towards body until slight discomfort is felt in back of thigh. Hold for 30 seconds. Dorsi-flex foot to increase stretch. Slowly return to starting position. Repeat for right leg.

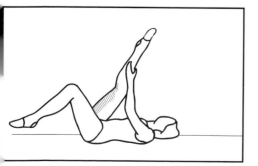

Figure 64: Hamstring stretch

Calf Stretch

Stand with one foot in front of the other (1m apart) with front leg bent and back leg straight. With feet firmly planted on the floor, push down on back leg and lower hips. Hold for 30 seconds; repeat with opposite leg.

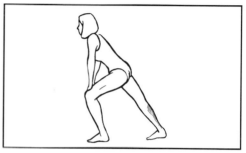

Figure 65: Calf stretch

Front Hip Stretch

Move right leg forward until knee is directly over ankle; knee of left leg should rest on floor. Keep both knees in this position, move front of hip down until slight discomfort is felt. Hold for 30 seconds. Slowly return to starting position. Repeat with opposite leg. Make sure knee of front leg is not in front of ankle, as this puts the knee joint into an unstable position and can cause injury.

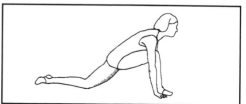

Figure 66: Front hip stretch

Groin Stretch

a   Lie on back and gently let knees part, soles of feet held together, until slight discomfort is felt. Hold for 30 seconds. Slowly return to the starting position. Repeat.

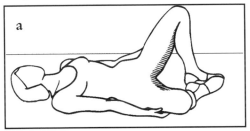

Figure 67: Basic groin stretch (a)

b   Sit with soles of feet together, rest elbows against knees as shown. Lean forward from hips until slight discomfort is felt in groin area. Hold for 30 seconds. Slowly return to starting position. Repeat. Care must be taken to bend from hips and not from spine. Eyes should be looking forward.

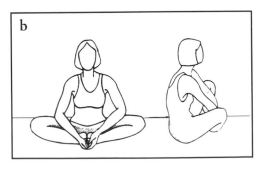

Figure 68: Intermediate groin stretch (b)

c   Sit with legs comfortably wide apart. Lean forward, bending from hips, until slight discomfort is felt on inside of legs. Hold for 30 seconds. Slowly return to starting position. Repeat. Ensure that bending occurs from hips only and eyes are looking forward. Remember always to keep back straight.

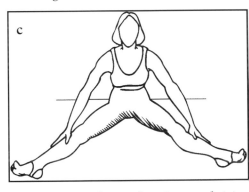

Figure 69: Advanced groin stretch (c)

Back, Shoulder, Forearm Stretch (Cat Stretch)

Reach arms forwards and extend spine, keeping head down. Concentrate on feeling stretch in broad back muscle. When a position of slight discomfort is reached, hold for 30 seconds.

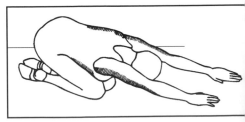

Figure 70: Cat stretch

> **Flexibility and the young performer:**
>
> - Children's immature bone structure means that the epiphyseal areas (ie bone-cartilage, bone-junctions) are especially susceptible to damage from over-stretching.
>
> - The use of external forces (gravity or forces from partners or coaches) to stretch beyond the point under the child's normal control should be avoided.
>
> - Children should be shown slow stretching exercises which remain solely under their own control.
>
> - Children should avoid ballistic exercises.
>
> - If performing any flexibility exercises, children should be well supervised and emphasis should be placed on sound technique.

6.9 Flexibility Assessment

Some coaches use flexibility tests to demonstrate improvement, increase motivation and provide objective feedback for training and competition. Unfortunately, the tests may give an inaccurate and relatively arbitrary set of values if not conducted correctly. It is important to avoid competition between individuals being tested, for this encourages the use of unsafe techniques to achieve a better score. Individuals should seek improvement from one testing occasion to another. Correct supervision and adherence to test protocols is essential. The essence of good flexibility work is slow, relaxed, gentle movements followed by relaxed holding of positions. As soon as assessment is introduced, relaxation becomes more difficult to maintain and results may not reflect flexibility as much as tension. There are various other variables which may affect the assessment:

- **The warmth of a performer's** muscles can affect the results obtained and it is not possible to be certain that each performer is equally well warmed-up. Maintaining the temperature of the testing environment will help.

- **The level of previous muscle activity** will affect results because exercise always creates some degree of fatigue. This in turn stimulates some unpredictable level of tension in the muscles.

- **A selection of sites should be tested** to achieve an overall indication of flexibility. The most common site used for testing is the hamstring muscle along with the more complex joints (eg back, shoulders and hips). Therefore, it becomes difficult to isolate the relevant movements and repeat the methods accurately.

- **A reduction in temperature** during the process may adversely affect the objectivity of the tests and lead to injury.

- **Static measurements** obtained by most flexibility tests may not relate to dynamic situations.

It must be remembered that the important coaching quality is to know (theoretically and practically) how to improve a performer's flexibility to achieve maximum potential. Probably the most significant assessment is to make subjective (but informed) judgements about the location of tensions and restrictions in the movements of the performers by using clear observations, assisted where possible and necessary by experienced and qualified observers of movement (eg sports scientists, physiotherapists, paediatricians and physical educationalists). This will identify areas that need more attention and then programmes can be devised to work on these areas.

Adequate preparation is needed prior to flexibility testing. This will include the initial mobility/pulse raising exercises (5–8 minutes) to prepare and warm the body, followed by continuous dynamic stretching where the body temperature must be maintained.

Specific flexibility exercises need to be chosen to reflect the sport or test. Think about the importance of maintaining body heat throughout. Performers develop efficient ways of dissipating excess heat by blood redistribution and sweating. However, this makes them vulnerable to cooling down quickly (eg at the end of an event or between tests). Appropriate safeguards are needed which may include warming-up again, a continuous circuit or the use of extra clothing.

6.10 Typical Flexibility Tests

The hamstring/lower back flexibility (sit and reach test), usually considered to be a good test of general flexibility, can be assessed by measurement and observation.

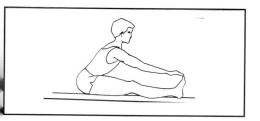

Figure 71: Sit and reach flexibility test

- Before conducting the test, it is important to warm-up thoroughly (especially the trunk, lower back and hamstrings).

- In a sitting position with the legs straight out in front, lean forward, keeping legs straight and toes pointing vertically upwards.

- Hold the head up and attempt to slide fingers towards the toes. If possible, place a metre rule alongside the inside of the leg and slide the fingers up the rule as far as possible while maintaining contact with the rule.

- Performers should not bounce or rock backwards and forwards to gain distance as this will affect the accuracy of the measurement and may cause injury. The furthest point reached should be measured.

Three attempts should be allowed and the best recorded. In most tests a measurement of 15cm or more would indicate good flexibility (eg being able to touch the toes and beyond), although this may not be the case if an individual has long legs and/or short arms.

TASK

It will help you to appreciate the factors affecting potential range of movement by carrying out the sit and reach test under different conditions. Try measuring your own flexibility and explain the differences in your results using the sit and reach test in different situations:

1 On waking while warm and relaxed.

2 After jogging or cycling for ten minutes.

3 After sitting for as long as possible, back against the wall, legs at right angles at knee.

4 When body is cold (do not force this stretch).

5 After ten minutes of hamstring stretches in the warm.

6.11 Fitting in Flexibility Training

It can be difficult to motivate performers to improve flexibility. There is a wide range of individual differences which can be discouraging to the less flexible performer. However, flexibility training can be included in everyday life as long as the principles of warm-up are remembered. Once the stretches have been learnt, individuals can incorporate them into daily activities (eg reading the paper while holding a groin stretch with legs apart, stretching while showering).

6.12 Summary

The importance of flexibility training in any sport is often ignored. This may be because it demands frequent, patient and repetitive work to produce relatively small gains. However, its overall contribution to performance enhancement and injury prevention is all too often underestimated. It is important that the knowledge gained from Chapters One and Two is applied when designing appropriate flexibility training programmes.

There are several other sources of information which will provide further details on flexibility:

Alter M (1998) **Sport stretch.** Champaign IL, Human Kinetics. ISBN 0 880118 23 7

Beaulieu, JE (1980) **Stretching for all sports.** Stanford CAL, Athletic Press. ISBN 0 87095 079 7

Hazeldine, R (2000) **Fitness for sport.** Marlborough, Crowood Press. (Chapter 4). ISBN 1 861263 36 8

McAtee, R (1999) **Facilitated stretching.** London, A & C Black. ISBN 0 736000 66 6

Norris C M (1994) **Flexibility: principles and practice.** London, A & C Black. ISBN 0 713640 37 5

Smith, Bob (1996) **Flexibility for sport.** Marlborough, Crowood Press. ISBN 1 852239 85 9

* Wilkinson, D and Moore, P (1995) **A guide to field based fitness testing.** Leeds, National Coaching Foundation. ISBN 0 947850 55 4

* Complimentary with the **sports coach UK** workshop *Field Based Fitness Testing* or available from **Coachwise 1st4sport** (tel 0113-201 5555 or visit www.1st4sport.com).

TASK

The tasks below can be used to test your understanding of flexibility and the structural limitations. This can be directly related to your specific sport to assist in designing appropriate training sessions and improving overall performance.

1 Identify the major joints used in your sport and the type of movement the joint allows. Identify the factors which limit the potential range of movement of these joints. Using this knowledge, reflect on past injuries you or others may have suffered in relation to joint structure. How can exercises be adapted in the future to avoid such injuries?

2 Analyse the flexibility exercises used in your sport. Are these appropriate to the muscle action involved? Does the warm-up and cool-down sequence contain adequate stretches covering all the muscle groups used in your sport? Adapt the programme to utilise developmental stretches fully to enhance effectiveness of the major muscle groups employed.

3 Work on your own flexibility for at least 30 minutes, five times a week for four weeks. Monitor and record improvements.

CONCLUSION

The information in this handbook is intended to help coaches, teachers and performers to understand the key issues which influence the development of physical fitness and reduce the likelihood of injury. It is important they recognise and respect the intricate structure and function of the body and seek effective and safe ways to develop the body's physiological potential in accordance with the specific demands of the sport. The handbook should have provided a valuable insight into the effects of training.

To continue to update and develop your coaching knowledge and skills, you are advised to take note of the workshops and resources recommended throughout the book. These will help to extend your knowledge further on specific topics and improve your coaching.

Recommended **sports coach UK** workshops and resources (complimentary with the corresponding workshop) include:

scUK Workshop	Accompanying Resource
A Guide to Mentoring Sports Coaches	A Guide to Mentoring Sports Coaches
Analysing your Coaching	Analysing your Coaching
Coaching and the Law	–
Coaching Children and Young People	Coaching Young Performers
Coaching Disabled Performers	Coaching Disabled Performers
Coaching Methods and Communication	The Successful Coach
Equity in Your Coaching	Equity in Your Coaching
Field-based Fitness Testing	A Guide to Field Based Fitness Testing
Fitness and Training	Physiology and Performance
Fuelling Performers	Fuelling Performers
Goal-setting and Planning	Planning Coaching Programmes
Good Practice and Child Protection	Protecting Children
Imagery Training	Imagery Training

scUK Workshop	Resource
Improving Practices and Skill	Improving Practices and Skill
Injury Prevention and Management	Sports Injury
Motivation and Mental Toughness	Motivation and Mental Toughness
Observation, Analysis and Video	Observation, Analysis and Video
Performance Profiling	Performance Profiling
The Responsible Sports Coach	–
Understanding Eating Disorders	–

Details of all **scUK** resources are available from:

Coachwise 1st4sport
Coachwise Ltd
Chelsea Close
Off Amberley Road
Armley
Leeds LS12 4HP
Tel: 0113-201 5555
Fax: 0113-231 9606

scUK also produces a technical journal, *Faster, Higher, Stronger (FHS)* Details of this service are available from:

sports coach UK
114 Cardigan Road
Headingley
Leeds LS6 3BJ
Tel: 0113-274 4802
Fax: 0113-275 5019
E-mail: coaching@sportscoachuk.org
Website: www.sportscoachuk.org

For direct bookings on **scUK** workshops, please contact:

Workshop Booking Centre
Chelsea Close
Off Amberley Road
Armley
Leeds LS12 4HP
Tel: 0845-601 3054
Fax: 0113-231 9606

For details of all **scUK** workshops, contact your nearest Regional Training Unit or home countries office or visit www.sportscoachuk.org. RTU contact details are available from **sports coach UK.**

a

b

c

Index